TOPICS FROM EPR RESEARCH

Edited by **Ahmed M. Maghraby**

Topics From EPR Research

http://dx.doi.org/10.5772/intechopen.75082

Edited by Ahmed M. Maghraby

Contributors

Sounik Kiran Kumar Dash, Taimoor Khan, Andrej Zorko, Betül Çalişkan, Ali Cengiz Çalişkan, Chryssoula Drouza, Smaragda Spanou, Anastasios D. Keramidas, Ahmed M. Maghraby

Notice

Statements and opinions expressed in the chapters are these of the individual contributors and not necessarily those of the editors or publisher. No responsibility is accepted for the accuracy of information contained in the published chapters. The publisher assumes no responsibility for any damage or injury to persons or property arising out of the use of any materials, instructions, methods or ideas contained in the book.

First published in London, United Kingdom, 2019 by IntechOpen

IntechOpen is the global imprint of INTECHOPEN LIMITED, registered in England and Wales, registration number: 11086078, The Shard, 25th floor, 32 London Bridge Street

London, SE19SG – United Kingdom

Printed in Croatia

British Library Cataloguing-in-Publication Data

A catalogue record for this book is available from the British Library

Additional hard copies can be obtained from orders@intechopen.com

Topics From EPR Research, Edited by Ahmed M. Maghraby

p. cm.

Print ISBN 978-1-78985-299-8

Online ISBN 978-1-78985-300-1

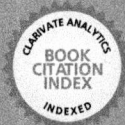

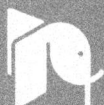

Meet the editor

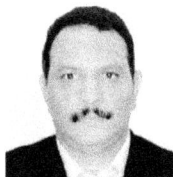

Ahmed M. Maghraby graduated from Cairo University, Faculty of Science, Egypt, in 1995 and started his career as a scientist at the National Institute of Standards, Egypt. He received his MSc degree in 1999 and his PhD degree from Cairo University in 2003 for the study of calibration and characterization of organic material for use in radiation dosimetry using electron paramagnetic resonance (EPR). In 1999, he worked as a guest researcher in the National Institute of Standards and Technology in Maryland, USA, and as a visiting scientist in Dartmouth College (EPR Center for the Study of Viable Systems) in New Hampshire, USA, in 2008. Also, he worked as a guest researcher in the Physikalisch-Technische Bundesanstalt, Germany's national metrology institute, in 2006. He has led and participated in several international research projects on radiation measurements. His research interest is in ionizing radiation metrology, especially ionization chambers, EPR, and thermoluminescence dosimetry. He is a reviewer for several peer-reviewed journals, has supervised a number of master's and PhD theses, and he has been elected as Vice-President of the National Committee of Physics in Egypt.

Contents

Preface VII

Chapter 1   **Introductory Chapter: Electron Paramagnetic Resonance 1**
Ahmed M. Maghraby

Chapter 2   **Biomedical EPR 5**
Betül Çalişkan and Ali Cengiz Çalişkan

Chapter 3   **Determination of Magnetic Anisotropy by EPR 23**
Andrej Zorko

Chapter 4   **EPR Methods Applied on Food Analysis 45**
Chryssoula Drouza, Smaragda Spanou and Anastasios D. Keramidas

Chapter 5   **Modeling of Dielectric Resonator Antennas using Numerical
Methods Applied to EPR 65**
Sounik Kiran Kumar Dash and Taimoor Khan

Preface

Electron paramagnetic resonance (EPR) (also called electron spin resonance) was first detected experimentally in Kazan by Zavoisky in 1945 [1] when he succeeded in detecting a radio-frequency absorption line from a hydrous copper chloride ($CuCl_2.2H_2O$) sample; the resonance line was detected at a magnetic field of 4.76 mT for a frequency of 133 MHz. After Zavoisky's discovery of EPR, many spectrometers were built in different places in the world and recording of EPR spectra of different materials was increased for different applications.

However, the story started earlier, when Stern and Gerlach proved that electron moment can take only discrete orientations despite the sphericity of the atom [2]. Shortly, Uhlenbeck and Goudsmit [3] linked the electron magnetic moment with the concept of electron spin angular momentum. Soon after Zavoisky's experiment, results were interpreted by Frankel [4]. Following World War II, complete microwave systems were available at low cost, which motivated research in the field of EPR. The first resonance spectra from organic free radicals were reported by Pake [5].

Nowadays, EPR spectroscopy is a very wide and rich field, which has many methods and many applications in different scientific disciplines. EPR applications extend from medicine and biology to dating and geology, passing through a wide spectrum of chemical and physical applications and studies.

Technologies employed for building EPR spectrometers are reflected on extreme microwave bands (frequencies) and huge magnets leading to the feasibility to monitor very subtle details compared to the early beginnings of EPR. The more achievements and progress in developing equipment and systems of EPR, the more applications arise and hence more secrets in the material under investigation can be uncovered.

In the current book, there are brief reviews of some selected topics related to EPR, highlighting in some way how far the progress on EPR has traveled since it was discovered seven decades ago.

The achievements in EPR techniques and equipment are expected to continue in the future to uncover more details of matters containing unpaired electrons and combining them in the form of useful information leading to increased welfare for humanity.

Prof. Dr. Ahmed M. Maghraby
Ionizing Radiation Metrology Laboratory
National Institute of Standards (NIS)
Egypt, Giza

References

[1] E. Zavoisky. 1945. "Spin-magnetic resonance in paramagnetics." J. Phys., USSR, 9, 211.

[2] W. Gerlach, O. Stern. 1921. "Der experimentelle Nachweis des magnetischen Moments des Silberatoms." Zeitschrift für Physik, 8, 110.

[3] G. Uhlenbeck, S. Goudsmit. 1925. "Ersetzung der Hypothese vom unmechanischen Zwang durch eine Forderung bezfiglich des inneren Verhaltens jedes einzelnen Elektrons." Naturwissenschaften, 13, 953.

[4] J. Frenkel. 1945. "On the theory of relaxation losses, connected with magnetic resonance in solid bodies." J. Phys. USSR, 9, 299.

[5] G. Pake, J. Townsend, S. Weissman. 1952. "Hyperfine structure in the paramagnetic resonance of the ion (SO3)2 NO–." Phys. Rev., 85, 682.

Chapter 1

Introductory Chapter: Electron Paramagnetic Resonance

Ahmed M. Maghraby

Additional information is available at the end of the chapter

http://dx.doi.org/10.5772/intechopen.83028

1. Introduction

Electron paramagnetic resonance (EPR) is similar to the nuclear magnetic resonance (NMR) where both of them describe the case of resonance of an atomic particle as a result of high-frequency electromagnetic radiation absorption in the presence of external magnetic field. The main difference is that NMR is related to nucleus, while EPR is related to the unpaired electron.

1.1. Basic concepts

The electron, as a charged rotating particle, possesses a magnetic field which makes the electron appears as a minute magnet [1]. In normal cases, for the unpaired electron (single electron), the spin energy levels are degenerate, and electrons spin randomly.

After applying an external magnetic field, spin energy levels split, and electrons spin either aligned to or opposite to the direction of the magnetic field. Splitting of the spin energy levels results in the emergence of some energy difference (ΔE); hence, electrons aligned parallel to the external magnetic field and occupying the lower energy level are more than those aligned antiparallel to the external magnetic field and occupying the upper energy level.

When incident photon energy (**hv**) matches the energy difference between the two energy levels, some electrons are excited in the upper energy level and flip their spin direction. After a time (t_1), the relaxation time, excited electrons return to their original state emitting photons whose energy is equal to ΔE.

Such process is expressed by the following formula:

$$hv = \Delta E = gBHM \tag{1}$$

---

where **h** is Planck's constant, **v** is the microwaves frequency, and **g** is the spectroscopic splitting factor: g_e = 2.002319304386(20), where g_e is the spectroscopic splitting factor for a free electron [2, 3].

B is Bohr magneton, B is the basic unit of a small magnet for an electron spin, **H** is the magnetic flux density of the external magnetic field, and **M** is the magnetic quantum number, **M**: M = ± ½. **Figure 1** represents the process of electron spin resonance (ESR).

1.2. Spectrometer structure

A conventional continuous wave (cw) spectrometer is represented in **Figure 2**. The figure is composed of four groups: the source components, the magnet system, the detection system, and the modulation system. The function of the first group, the source, is to produce the electromagnetic radiation and holds the sample to be subjected to the incident waves. The source region also controls and directs the incident microwaves. The magnet system helps to provide the required magnetic field necessary for splitting the energy level; the field must be homogeneous and stable over the desired range. Both of the modulation system and the detection system act to amplify the received signal and to record it [3].

1.3. High-field high-frequency measurements

Usually, EPR measurements are carried out at X-band and Q-band due to the instrumental availability, where conventional electromagnets can provide up to 1 Tesla. However, higher spectral resolution needs led to the use of more advanced EPR measurements with higher microwave bands and more intensive magnets. Currently, there are many bands for EPR measurements according to the practical requirements. **Table 1** represents different microwave frequencies and the corresponding values for magnetic field [4, 5].

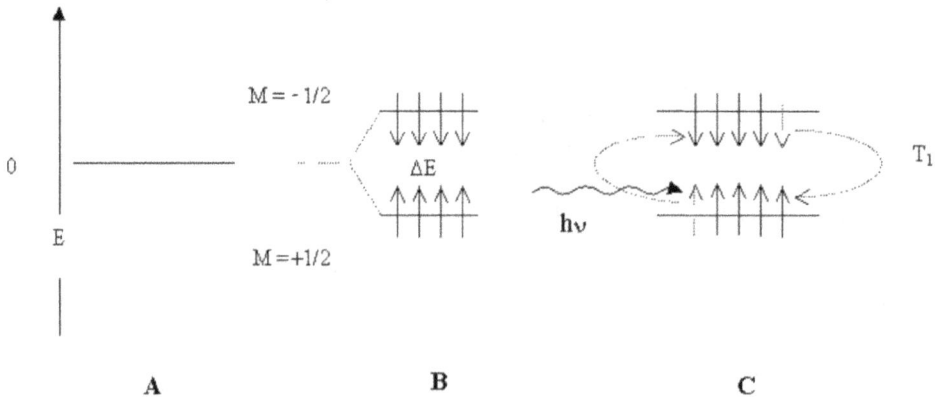

Figure 1. (A) No applied magnetic field and no spin levels splitting. (B) Energy separation of an unpaired electron spin under a magnetic field (Zeeman effect). (C) Flipping of spins by microwave absorption and flopping of spins within the spin-lattice relaxation time, T_1.

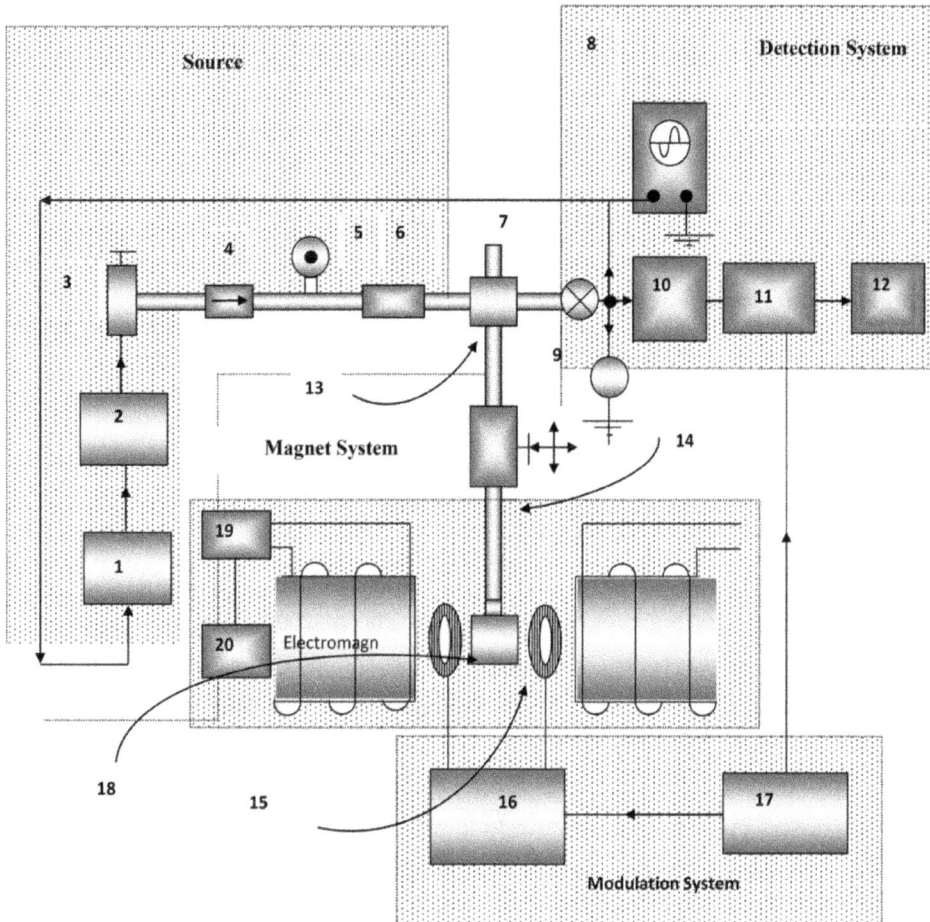

Figure 2. Block diagram of a typical X-band EPR spectrometer employing 100 kHz phase-sensitive detection. (1) Automatic frequency control. (2) Microwave source power supply. (3) Microwave source (klystron or Gunn diode). (4) Isolator. (5) Frequency counter. (6) Attenuator. (7) Terminating load. (8) Oscilloscope. (9) Detector crystal. (10) 100 kHz signal amplifier. (11) 100 kHz signal detector. (12) Pen recorder and data bank (or computer). (13) Circular or hybrid tee. (14) Cavity system. (15) 100 kHz modulation coils. (16) 100 kHz power amplifier. (17) 100 kHz oscillator. (18) Resonant cavity. (19) Magnet power supply. (20) Field scan drive [3].

Waveband	L	S	C	X	P	K	Q	U	V	E	W	F	D
λ/mm	300	100	75	30	20	12.5	8.5	6	4.6	4	3.2	2.7	2.1
ν/GHz	1	3	4	10	15	24	35	50	65	75	95	111	140
H/T	0.03	0.11	0.14	0.33	0.54	0.86	1.25	1.8	2.3	2.7	3.5	3.9	4.9

Table 1. Different microwave bands and the corresponding magnetic field.

The higher the frequency is used, the more intensive magnetic field is needed to reach the resonance. High-field high-frequency measurements can provide more detailed spectra and hence more molecular information.

Author details

Ahmed M. Maghraby

Address all correspondence to: maghrabism@yahoo.com

Ionizing Radiation Dosimetry Department, National Institute of Standards (NIS), Giza, Egypt

References

[1] Philip Rieger H. Electron Spin Resonance. Analysis and Interpretation. Vol. 104. The Royal Society of Chemistry. Annual Reports on the Progress of Chemistry, Section C: Physical Chemistry, Springer Nature Singapore Pte Ltd. 2007. pp. 81-123

[2] Nakagawa K, Eaton GR, Eaton SS. Electron spin relaxation times of irradiated alanine. International Journal of Radiation Applications and Instrumentation. Part A. Applied Radiation and Isotopes. 1993;44:73-77

[3] Weil JA, Bolton JR, Wertz JE. Electron Paramagnetic Resonance, Elementary Theory and Practical Applications. New York: A Wiley-Interscience Publication, John Wiley & Sons, Inc; 1994

[4] Brustolon M, Giamello E. Electron Paramgnetic Resonance: A Practitioner's Toolkit. New York: John Wiley & Sons, Inc; 2009

[5] Eaton GR, Eaton SS, Barr DP, Weber RT. Quantitative EPR. Wien: Springer-Verlag; 2010

Chapter 2

Biomedical EPR

Betül Çalişkan and Ali Cengiz Çalişkan

Additional information is available at the end of the chapter

http://dx.doi.org/10.5772/intechopen.79271

Abstract

Free radicals may participate in biological processes. An enzymatic dehydrogenation involved free radical intermediates. The oxidations of organic molecules, although they are bivalent, proceed in two successive steps, the intermediate state being a free radical. In an attempt to correlate the action of such a variety of carcinogenic agents as sodium hydroxide, ultraviolet and ionizing radiations and thousands of organic compounds, a free radical intermediate always suggests itself. Electron paramagnetic resonance (EPR) has brought sufficient sensitivity and discrimination to observe free radical intermediates directly in many of these reactions. EPR is aided by an increased sensitivity in many cases and has made a much greater contribution by distinguishing among paramagnetic ions, odd molecules and free radicals.

Keywords: electron paramagnetic resonance (EPR), free radical, paramagnetic ion, oxidation, organic molecule, enzymatic dehydrogenation, carcinogenic agent

1. Introduction

Biomedical application of EPR has gained momentum in recent times. All atoms and molecules cannot be studied by EPR technique. Atoms and molecules with electronic magnetic moment and angular momentum can be studied with this method. Four classes of compounds with biological properties stand out in EPR studies:

a. odd molecules and free radicals,

b. biradicals,

c. triplet electronic states and

d. transition element ions.

In these, single molecules and free radicals can occur biologically in the following situations: univalent redox reactions, enzymatic oxidizations (dehydrogenations), radiation damage and photosynthesis. The biomedical application of electron paramagnetic resonance (EPR) has been grouped together under five headings:

a. The study of free radicals in living tissue.

b. The relation between free radicals and carcinogenic activity.

c. The study of oxidation-reduction systems and enzyme interaction.

d. Photosynthesis and optical absorption studies.

e. X-irradiation of biological material.

2. The EPR study of free radicals in living tissue

The first study of free radical concentration in living tissues by EPR was conducted by Commoner et al. [1]. The presence of water in biological materials poses difficulties in EPR studies. The interaction of the large dipole moment with the microwave electric field in the liquid phase causes a large quenching and a Q factor decrease. This can be corrected using smaller samples (e.g. sample tubes of 1-mm diameter instead of the normal 5-mm diameter). Working with a high radiofrequency instead of microwaves region can be useful to obtain high sensitivity for aqueous studies. The loss due to the dipole interaction falls with a decreasing frequency. At lower frequencies, a larger volume should be used to increase sensitivity. Such a situation is suitable for free radical concentration studies.

If the experiments are carried out in the microwave area, the loss from water can be removed by freezing the sample and by making the measurements at liquid nitrogen temperatures, or by freezing and drying the material before it is placed in the cavity. Radicals can be adversely affected in both methods. In this case, studies with smaller sample tubes should be preferred at room temperature. Commoner et al. [1] prepared their first samples by free-drying by taking them from many different tissues. Thus, the powder samples were run on an X-band EPR spectrometer. The first results are given in **Table 1**. In metabolically active tissues such as green leaves, liver and kidney, it was noticed that there was a higher content of free radicals. In addition, the free radical concentration was found to be associated with protein components. It has also been shown by fractionation experiments that protein denaturation destroys the radical concentration.

According to the results obtained from studies done with ungerminated and germinated seeds and with leaves exposed to varying amounts of illumination, increasing the free radical concentration is associated with a high metabolic activity. For this reason, although no measurable free radical concentration was found in samples prepared from digitalis seeds before germination, a free radical concentration of 10^{-7} moles/g was obtained from the seeds obtained by the emergence of the primary root.

Material	Radical concentration (10^{-8} mole/g of dry weight)
Nicotiana tabacum, leaf	65
Nicotiana tabacum, roots	10
Coleus, leaf	180
Barley, leaf	25
Digitalis, germinating seeds	10
Carrot, root	8
Beet, root	6
Rabbit, blood	25
Rabbit, muscle	20
Rabbit, brain	25
Rabbit, liver	60
Rabbit, lung	30
Rabbit, heart	35
Rabbit, kidney	55
Frog, eggs	200
Drosophila, entire	4

Table 1. Radical concentration in different tissues.

These radical concentrations are associated with proteins, reach concentrations varying according to the level of metabolic activity and have the magnitudes consistent with the total electron-transporting content of the tissues [2].

Commoner et al. [1] identified the presence of a high free radical concentration in melanin, a pigmentation found in various biological tissues, Melanin formation in animals by UV or ionizing radiation [3]. This is evidence that free radical production takes place with irradiation of living tissue.

3. EPR study of free radicals and carcinogenic activity

Some researchers have acknowledged that free radicals participate in carcinogenic activity [4, 5]. Lipkin et al. [5] suggested that the carcinogenic activities of some large ring structures, together with mild reductive agents, could create negative ion-free radicals. Non-carcinogenic hydrocarbons, such as naphthalene, have also been shown to require very strong reducing agents before such radicals can be formed. Electron paramagnetic resonance is a powerful technique to test the accuracy of these findings.

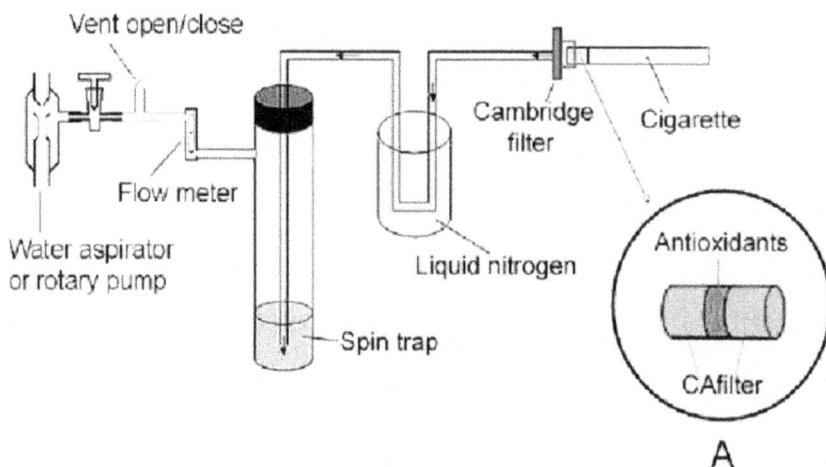

Figure 1. An apparatus for trapping cigarette smoke at low temperatures.

Several experiments have recently been carried out on the radical concentration in cigarette smoke [6]. The arrangement in which the cigarettes are fixed to a filter pump [7] is shown in **Figure 1**. Existing active radicals remain unchanged in the frozen state in the apparatus. After the freezing process is done, when the tube and the contents are processed in the EPR spectrometer for the radical concentration measurement process, it is possible to differentiate between short-lived active radicals and stabilizing radicals.

The concentration of radicals obtained in the frozen smoke condensate before warming was of the order of 10^{15} free electrons per gram. It should be noted that this condensate contains large amounts of solid carbon dioxide and ice. On warming, the condensate separated into an aqueous and an organic or a tarry phase. No radical concentration at all could be detected in the aqueous phase, and that in the organic phase was reduced by a factor of approximately six. The radicals that could still be detected in the latter were found to be highly stabilized, and no diminution of their concentration was found after several days. It would therefore appear from these experiments that the tar constituents of cigarette smoke contain about 6×10^{15} free electron/gram. Some of these radicals, being relatively short-lived, disappear when the condensate is warmed to 60°C for some minutes. The remainder, however, appears to be very stable and long-lived. It is probable that these stable radicals are very similar to those formed by pyrolysis of other organic matter.

These experiments therefore show that there is a relatively high concentration of both active and stabilized free radicals in cigarette smoke when it is first formed, and it is possible that either or both of these might act as carcinogenic agents. It is important to note in this connection that most bioassays in tobacco carcinogenesis have been carried out using relatively old condensates, and it is now evident that these will be deficient in the unstable free radicals initially present in the smoke.

The subject of carcinogenesis still needs to be resolved and understood. When the effects of various carcinogenic agents such as sodium hydroxide, ultraviolet and ionizing radiation and thousands of organic compounds are examined, a free radical intermediate always plays a role. Although there is no direct evidence to date, smog studies and recent work by Lyons et al. [6] have found that soot and tobacco smoke contain highly active radicals and signaled possible links with lung cancer.

The concentration of stable free radicals in atmospheric soot is about 100 times larger than in cigarette smoke, but as with the polycyclic hydrocarbons [8], adsorption on comparatively larger particles and further stabilization as a result are likely to render them inaccessible to the cells. It is evident that a large amount of systematic work will have to be performed before the correlation between free radical concentration and carcinogenic activity is established, but these initial experiments show that electron resonance should be of considerable help in these studies.

4. EPR study of oxidation: reduction and enzyme systems

It has already been seen that free radicals have been postulated as necessary intermediates in biological oxidation-reduction systems [9] and that the preliminary measurements of Commoner et al. [1] appear to support this hypothesis. Free radical processes have also been postulated as taking part in most enzyme reactions [10], and kinetic studies often show that chain processes are present. A large number of electron resonance studies of enzyme reactions are now in progress to investigate the details of these reaction mechanisms. At the time of writing, no detailed results on actual enzyme systems have been published, but some preliminary basic work on simpler oxidation-reduction systems has been reported.

One series of organic compounds closely related to biologically important molecules are the phthalocyanines. These are large planar molecules consisting of a conjugated ring system very similar to that of the porphyrin ring and containing either two protons or a divalent metal atom at the center. If these are oxidized by such agents as ceric sulfate, a two-stage oxidation process takes place via a transient intermediate stage which often gives the solution a markedly different color for a few seconds. There has been considerable speculation [11] as to whether this intermediate oxidation stage involved a change of valency of the central metal atom or the liberation of an unpaired electron in the ring system. Electron resonance studies are able to give a very direct answer to such a problem as this, since different valence states of the central metal atom will have characteristic g-values well displaced from the free-spin value, whereas a mobile electron in the ring system will have a narrow 'free radical' resonance line very close to $g = 2.0$.

It was found experimentally [12] that all the phthalocyanines studied had intermediate oxidation states that gave a narrow resonance line with a g-value very close to that of a free spin. This was therefore conclusive proof that the oxidation process involved mobile electrons in the conjugated ring system. In some cases [12], it was possible to follow the oxidation process through its different stages and watch the growth and decay of the intermediate on the oscilloscope of the resonance spectrometer.

Another oxidation system of considerable biological importance is the oxidation of ferrihemoglobin to its metastable state. This system has been studied in some detail [13, 14] by electron resonance. The systematic analysis of these results is a good illustration of the fact that it is important to consider all possible interactions when investigating biological systems. As in the case of the phthalocyanines, the oxidation intermediate will either involve an unpaired electron in the conjugated ring system or a change in the valency state of the central iron atom. Chemical investigations [15] give inconclusive evidence as to which of these mechanisms is actually present.

In the initial electron resonance studies [13], it was found that a strong narrow free radical line with a g-value of 2.0023 was obtained; methemoglobin or metmyoglobin was oxidized by hydrogen peroxide or periodate. By analogy with the results obtained from the phthalocyanines, it was therefore assumed that the oxidation involved electron removal from the π-orbitals of the porphyrin ring. Furthermore detailed and systematic investigations of this system [14] confirmed that there is a close connection between the free radical and the peroxide compound, as shown by four separate sets of results. First, the formation of the free radical is specific for the methemoglobin peroxide reaction, since it does not occur in model systems such as serum albumin-Fe-H_2O_2 or metmyoglobin cyanide-Fe-H_2O_2. Secondly, the removal of excess peroxide by catalase does not affect the free radical. Thirdly, the amount of free radical is proportional to the initial concentration of metmyoglobin, under comparable conditions. Fourthly, the free radical is destroyed by substances reducing the peroxide compound (ferrocyanide, nitrite, iodide, p-cresol).

In spite of the above conclusions, however, there are further results which show that the free radical cannot be identified with the peroxide compound itself. The reasons for this can be summarized as follows. First, the calculated concentration of free radical in most favorable case was only 9% of the peroxide compound. Secondly, its concentration varied widely under conditions in which the amount of peroxide compound remained approximately constant. Thus, an increase of pH from 6 to 10 decreased the free radical concentration by 80%, while the peroxide compound was formed equally well at these pH values. Thirdly, the preaddition of stoichiometric quantities of ferrocyanide to the metmyoglobin before the formation of peroxide compound almost eliminated the free radical. Such treatment has been found [15] to remove the first oxidizing equivalent of hydrogen peroxide lost during the formation of the peroxide compound.

These experiments therefore suggest that the free radical is not the peroxide compound itself, but a product of oxidation by the first oxidizing equivalent, which is likely to be a hydroxyl radical [15]. The free radical signal is thus probably due to oxidation of part of the globin molecule, and although it takes place at the same time as the peroxide compound is formed, it is not associated directly with this oxidation mechanism. It is nevertheless of considerable interest as it is an example of a reversible univalent oxidation state in a biological system which does not involve valence changes of a transition metal. The fact that the formation of the actual peroxide compound involved a change in the binding of the iron atom was demonstrated conclusively by observing the metmyoglobin resonance at g = 6.0 [16] as oxidation occurred. This resonance was found to decrease as the peroxide compound was formed, indicating a change from ionic to covalent binding [17] as the oxidation took place.

It may be noted in this connection that a detailed study of the different derivatives of hemoglobin by electron resonance not only allows the actual orbitals involved in the binding to be determined [17] but also gives detailed structural information on the porphyrin and histidine planes [16–20].

This work on the oxidation states of hemoglobin and myoglobin indicates the necessity for careful systematic studies if the electron resonance spectra of these biological systems are to be correctly interpreted. This remark will apply with an even greater force to the catalase and peroxidase [14] and other complex enzyme systems that are being currently investigated.

It may be noted that a kinetic study of these enzyme reactions not only allows the variation of free radical concentration to be followed but also enables correlations to be made between this and the concentration of any paramagnetic atoms that are present. The exact role of different metallic ions in enzyme reactions has been a matter of speculation for some time, and in some cases, they are assumed to play an essential step in the oxidation-reduction mechanism, and in others, they appear to enter only as impurities. If the concentration of the metallic ions is monitored [21] at the same time as that of the free radicals, these effects can be clearly distinguished.

The idea that free radicals can participate in biological processes has recently been explored. It has been suggested by Haber and Willstatter [22] that free radical intermediates form a large part of the enzymatic dehydrogenations. In the single electron transfer hypothesis of biological oxidation, most of the reactants in metabolic redox systems are double molecules. In this case, all the electrons in these molecules are found in pairs. Thus, it is considered that all of the electron transfers must be in pairs. In the two-electron transfer, certain molecules must be present which proceed by a one-electron step. An example of this is the process of delivering an electron under oxidation or reduction to metallo-organic substances of cytochrome. It has been suggested by Michaelis that all the oxidation of organic molecules proceeds in two successive stages and that free radical is an intermediate state [23]. Michaelis proved this experimentally.

Spectrophotometric kinetic studies have shown that various biologically active substances such as free radicals are present as intermediates between fully reduced and fully oxidized states. Prior to the discovery of the electron paramagnetic resonance technique, static susceptibility measurements have been a direct method of detecting more than 10^{-6} moles of paramagnetic molecule solution. Brill [24] has recently successfully carried out an experiment that can detect a 10^{-7} molar solution of paramagnetic molecules. However, Pauling and Coryell [25] gave many values for the magnetic susceptibility of hemoglobin. The hypothesis of Michaelis was not confirmed with complete success due to this low sensitivity. Thus, EPR has greatly contributed to the distinction between paramagnetic ions, odd molecules and free radicals through increased sensitivity.

There are many EPR studies related to non-enzymatic reduction of quinone and quinoid compounds [26]. Two consecutive one-electron transfers occur in these compounds. Furthermore, the lifetime of paramagnetic semi-quinone radicals depends on the isomeric form which is compatible with the differences in oxidation potentials and pH of the solution. While the free radical generated by the dehydrogenation of the hydroxyl group is stabilized in the alkaline solution, the free radical generated by the dehydrogenation of the amino group is stabilized in the acid solution. The compounds which give free radical concentrations are as follows:

p-benzoquinone, o-benzoquinone, catechol, pyrogallol, gallic acid, guaiacol, arsinol, resorcinol, 4-ethyl resorcinol, 4-propyl resorcinol, 4-butyl resorcinol, 4-amyl resorcinol, 4-hexyl resorcinol, 2-nitro resorcinol, gentisic acid, homogentisic acid, polyporic acid, tocopherol, 1,5

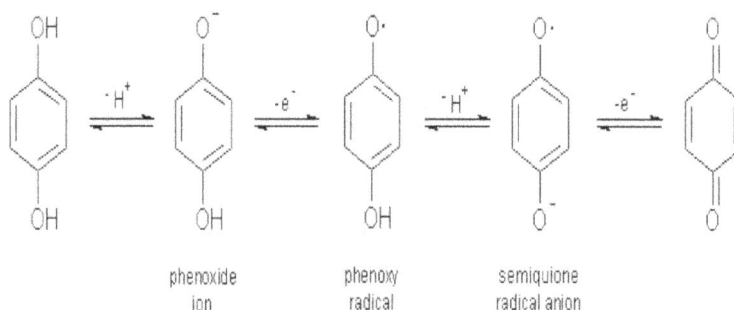

phenoxide
ion

phenoxy
radical

semiquione
radical anion

Figure 2. Quinone-hydroquinone redox reaction.

naphthalenediol, 1,4 naphthoquinone, 1,2 naphthoquinone, juglone, menedione, vitamin K_1, vitamin E, phthiocol, anthraquinone, anthraquinone β-sulphonic acid, alizarin, carminic acid, phenanthrene quinone, phenolphthalein, ascorbic acid, nicotinic acid, p-phenylene diamine, p-aminophenol, benzidine, diacetyl, benzil, ninhydrin, riboflavin, FMN, indigo, adrenaline.

If the lifetime of the free radical intermediate such as the parabenzoquinone redox reaction shown in **Figure 2** is short, the probability of a polymeric reaction is reduced.

Beinert [27], Commoner et al. [28] and Ehrenberg and Ludwig [29] conducted a number of studies on EPR studies of free radicals resulting from enzymatic oxidation-reduction reactions. Beinert has shown that the EPR signals observed for flavin enzyme and fatty acyl (CoA) dehydrogenase are associated with the re-oxidation of the enzyme-substrate complex by molecular oxygen [27]. However, more studies should be done to determine whether they will be confronted with other double flavin enzymes. Beinert could be shown by comparison with optical kinetics that the radicals observed in a single flavin enzyme and cytochrome reductase are intermediates in the enzyme substrate reaction itself.

In enzyme chemistry, the detection of paramagnetic ions in enzymatic reactions is important. In this subject, EPR plays an important role. Bray et al. [30] investigated the role of molybdenum in xanthine oxidase reactions, despite the oxidation state; Malmstrom et al. [31] investigated the role of Mn^{++} in enolase reactions; Malmstrom et al. [32] investigated the role of Cu^{++} in laccase; Beinert and Sands [33] investigated the role of Cu^{++} in cytochrome oxidase and the role of Fe^{++} in cytochrome-reductase [34]. In addition, after all the iron reduction (28 per cent), Beinert and Sands [33] showed that no free radical signal reduced by DPNH was produced. Because DPN shows a reaction sequence in which the electron flow sequence progresses in the form of substrate→flavin→iron. The answer to whether or not the iron is in contact with other electron receivers can only give EPR.

5. EPR studies on photosynthesis and optical absorption

The free radicals play an important role in photosynthesis, and it had been proposed previously that the excitation of chlorophyll during photosynthesis involved mono- [9] or bi-radical [35] formation. In the initial experiments [1], the leaves were lyophilized before insertion into the cavity, and hence kinetic studies on the specimens were not possible. In a more recent series of experiments, however, Commoner, Heise and Townsend [36] were able to study aqueous suspensions of chloroplasts, in situ in the cavity, under different conditions of illumination. This was achieved by the use of very small specimen tubes in conjunction with a high-sensitivity 100-kc/s field modulation spectrometer.

The chloroplasts, which are known to be responsible for the essential steps of photosynthesis [35], were prepared from leaves of *Nicotiana tabacum* by gentle hand maceration in an ice bath in a buffer solution of pH 8. After filtration and centrifugation, the chloroplasts were resuspended in 55% sucrose and stored in the cold. The spectrometer employed a reflection-type cavity and had a 2-mm diameter hole in the shorting end through which the light from a car headlamp was focused. In this way, the free radical concentration in the chloroplast suspension could be studied under different conditions of illumination, and the rate of growth and decay was measured accurately.

It was found that there was only a very small radical concentration in the absence of any illumination, but that this increased by about sixfold as soon as the 50 c.p. headlamp was switched on. Rapid tracing of the signal enabled an accurate plot of the growth of radical concentration to be obtained. It was found that the concentration rose exponentially to a steady value after the onset of illumination with an exponential time constant of 12 s. The decay of radical concentration when the lamp was switched off was also of an exponential form, but with a somewhat longer constant of 45 s. These results show conclusively that a steady-state radical concentration was being measured and not a system of trapped or stabilized radicals.

The variation of radical concentration with intensity and the wavelength of the incident illumination were also studied [36]. The concentration was found to rise with an increasing intensity but reached a saturation value at high levels, and this is also true of the photosynthetic activity of both chloroplasts and whole cells. It was also shown that the free radical concentration was produced by the same wavelength range 4000–7000 Å, which is responsible for photosynthesis. These experiments therefore provide conclusive evidence that one-electron intermediates with unstable molecular configurations are produced during photosynthetic reactions.

Further measurements on illuminated chloroplasts were then made by Sogo et al. [37]. In particular, they studied the variation of radical rise and decay time with the temperature of the specimen. Their results are summarized in **Table 2**, and the most striking feature of these results is that the signal growth time is approximately the same when the chloroplasts are frozen at −140°C as when they are at room temperature. This fact would appear to rule out the ordinary enzymatic oxidation-reduction reactions as the free radical intermediates in photosynthesis. The longer decay time at −140°C also suggests that excitation to the triplet state is not responsible for the observed signal, and it is unlikely that this would be observed in any case. It would therefore seem that the intermediate associated with photosynthesis is some form of electron produced by a dissociated bond or trapped in a quasi-crystalline lattice. It is noticeable [37] in this connection that the lines at room temperature show evidence

Substance	Light intensity (quanta/ sec.)	Temperature (°C)	Signal growth time	Signal decay time
Dried leaves	10^{15}	25	Minutes	Hours
Dried whole chloroplasts	10^{15}	25	Minutes	Hours
		60	Seconds	Seconds
Wet whole chloroplast	10^{15}	25	Seconds	1 minute
		−140	Seconds	Hours
Wet small chloroplast fragments	10^{15}	25	Seconds	Minutes
Wet large chloroplast fragments	10^{15}	24	30 s	30 s
	10^{16}	25	6 s	30 s
	10^{16}	−140	10 s	Hours

Table 2. Growth and decay time of radical concentration in photosynthesis material.

of exchange narrowing, but are wider at the lower temperatures, indicating a reduced mobility of the unpaired electrons.

Tollin and Calvin [38] have also performed detailed studies of the luminescence of similar chloroplast samples and have correlated these results with the electron resonance measurements. As a result of this, it would appear that the hypothesis of electron trapping and the production of holes is the most plausible theory of photosynthetic reaction. This semi-conductor theory of chloroplast action has been proposed by several investigators [39, 40] and is also supported by glow-curve and resistance measurements [40]. In this theory, the luminescence that occurs immediately after illumination ceases will be largely due to radiative recombination of nearly free electrons and holes. Following this, the thermal excitation of electrons and holes from the shallowest traps will produce further emission, and the decay constant will be a function of the trap depth and the temperature. The close correlation of the luminescence and electron resonance is explained in this way, and also the much longer decay times obtained at low temperatures, when the thermal excitation energy is much smaller while the trap depth remains more or less the same.

These initial electron resonance studies of photosynthesis are only of a preliminary nature, however, and the interpretation of the results must still be considered as somewhat speculative. They do illustrate very well, however, the kind of information that can be obtained, and the technique should prove to be a very powerful complement to all the normal luminescence and phosphorescence studies.

Photosynthesis, the biochemical process in which photoenergy transforms into chemical energy, involves steps of oxidation reduction. Thus, EPR is one of the important methods that clarify the photosynthesis process. Calvin and Sogo [41] and Commoner et al. [28] observed light-sensitive EPR signals on the chlorophyll system. Other important work in this regard was carried out by Sogo et al. [37] and Tollin and Calvin [38].

6. EPR study of X-irradiation of biological material

A study of the breakdown processes that occur in living tissue as a result of X- or γ-ray irradiation is one of the most important problems in modern medical physics. Electron resonance is one of the most direct and sensitive methods of investigation in this particular field, and the initial results have already shown that a large variety of different spectra can be obtained from different specimens. The energy of the incident quanta is not only great enough to break a very large number of different bonds but the secondary radical and non-radical species can also produce further change in the cell structure. Thus, most biological specimens contain a large percentage of water, and it is known that the OH˙ radicals formed in this by primary photolysis will combine and produce relatively high concentrations of hydrogen peroxide. This is very toxic for a large number of cellular reactions and may easily produce breakdown processes, the products of which can then be further attacked by primary or secondary radicals. Deductions of the mode of breakdown from the observed electron resonance spectra should therefore be made very tentatively until all possible mechanisms have been considered.

Electron resonance studies of this kind can be divided into two broad categories:

a. quantitative studies of free radical production as a function of radiation dosage and

b. qualitative analysis of the types of radical structure formed in the breakdown process.

In quantitative studies, it is possible to study either the dynamic concentrations which are formed in situ in the resonator, or the larger concentrations obtained in a solid or a viscous medium by a suitable trapping technique. In order to obtain dynamic concentrations of sufficient intensity, it is necessary to employ very powerful radiation sources, and this often requires pulse techniques. The use of pulsed irradiation can also give useful additional information. Thus, it is possible, in principle, to trigger the electron resonance spectrometer at a specified time delay after the irradiation pulse and hence obtain a series of measurements on the free radical decay between successive pulses. A high sensitivity detection with long-time constants is not feasible under such conditions, however, and this is another reason why high radiation dosages must be employed. Several laboratories are working on systems suitable for these quantitative dynamic studies, but to date, most information has come from the qualitative analysis of the different radical structures present in the breakdown process.

The identification of different radical species from the hyperfine pattern of their electron resonance spectra has been considered at some length. It was seen there that is often possible to pick out the presence of specific groups in the presence of other free radicals, and this method of analysis can now be extended to the more complex biological compounds. The results of Gordy et al. [40] on X-irradiated cystine and various fibrous proteins may be taken as a specific example of this. The electron resonance spectra of cystine, hair, nail and feather are obtained [42], and they are seen to be very similar. This similarity is even more striking when it is found that the spectra are not symmetrically placed around $g = 2$ and have splittings that vary with the strength of the external field. It would therefore appear that in each case, the free radicals must have an unpaired electron strongly localized on a sulfur or an oxygen atom with an associated anisotropic g-factor. It is noticeable in this connection that the spectra are very similar to those obtained from frozen solutions of sulfur in oleum [42].

Gordy et al. [43] in fact explain these spectra as due to an unpaired electron localized on the S-S bond of the cystine. Thus, if an electron is ejected by the irradiation from some point in the molecule, the vacancy probably moves to the S atoms to form an additional lower energy three-electron bond.

There is thus now a hole shared by the two sulfur atoms through exchange of their electrons, and the loss of an electron from the sulfur lone pair orbitals tends to strengthen rather than weaken the bond in this case.

From the marked similarity of the spectra of the irradiated hair, feather and toe-nail, it would appear that the radicals in these proteins must also be associated with their cystine content. The above hypothesis also explains why only the cystine spectrum is observed although the cystine group is a small fraction of the total amino acid content of the protein. If the three-electron S—S bond represents a lower energy state, the cystine is likely to donate an unpaired electron to any other ionized group formed by the irradiation. In this way, the two sulfur atoms of the cystine molecule act as an electron reservoir and supply electrons to fill vacancies at other points in the protein molecule, and such a mechanism should very much reduce the damage produced by the irradiation. It is therefore evident that in these particular cases, the electron resonance spectra have not only shown that the cystine type grouping is present in these proteins, but have also indicated that the breakdown process is transferred to the S—S bond, and molecular fracture is therefore not so likely to take place in these compounds.

These results indicate the type of reasoning that is used when deducing radiation effects from resonance spectra of complex molecules. Another example is given by the spectra observed from irradiated glycylglycine, silk, cattle hide and fish scale [43]. A symmetrical doublet with a frequency-independent splitting of 12 gauss is obtained in all of these cases. This is attributed to the direct dipole-dipole interaction between the hydrogen bonding proton and the unpaired electron localized on an oxygen atom of the adjacent polypeptide chain.

This method of analysis by 'correlation of similar spectra' will have to be employed in most of the biological studies in the immediate future. The conclusions deduced in this way must be considered as tentative and often as just one possible explanation among several others. As further results are obtained, however, a greater background of information will be built up on the most likely type of hyperfine interaction present in any particular system.

Gordy et al. [44, 45] have started a series of measurements on the electron resonance spectra observed from various X-irradiated proteins, to try and build up some systematic data for this purpose. With this in mind, the simpler peptide and polypeptides were studied first [44], so that their spectra could then be compared with those obtained from the more complex proteins. These investigations included X-irradiated glycylglycylglycine, DL-alanyl-DL-alanine, acetyl-DL-alanine, glycyl-DL-valine, acetyl-DL-leucine, and DL-alanylglycylglycine. The electron resonance spectra of the more complex proteins such as histone, insulin, hemoglobin and albumin were then investigated [45] and compared with those of the simpler proteins. It was found that two types of pattern were obtained in each case. One of these is very similar to that obtained from the irradiated cystine, and the other is a doublet similar to that obtained from the irradiated glycylglycine. It would therefore appear that the electron-donating power of the S-S bonds and the hydrogen bonding across the polypeptide chains may be general features in most protein structures. The work is also being extended to irradiated hormones and vitamins [44] such as progesterone parathyroid, vitamin A, vitamin K, ascorbic acid and also to irradiated nucleic acids [45] such as DNA, RNA, adenosine, cytidine and inosine. These measurements are all of a preliminary nature at the moment, and much careful and systematic work will have to be done before any definite conclusions can be established. The field is a very wide one, however, and when sufficient systematic measurements have been made, some detailed information on the different mechanisms associated with irradiation damage should emerge.

Free radical reactions in a biological system are controlled by both pH and antioxidants. The effect of antioxidants on radiation damage in the biological system is a known fact. Contrary to this effect, it is formed by sensitizers, which are good oxidants. The best examples are O_2 and quinones. In addition, various organic compounds can form active free radicals after reduction. An experiment showing free radical production as a secondary process in radiation damage can be summarized as follows: water and a mixture of 3% alcohol-riboflavin were reduced to 10^{-5} M riboflavin by ethyl alcohol radicals, resulting from OH and H radicals generated by 650 kV X-rays. This experiment was performed by Gordy et al. [43]. Information on the level of antioxidant can be obtained by titrating against a standard free radical solution and using EPR. Quantitative determinations of reduced free radical and therefore antioxidant concentrations are described by Blois et al. [46]. At this point, it is necessary to make more detailed studies on the clinical applications of EPR. EPR spectroscopy allows the observation of free radical intermediates in vivo. Commoner et al. [1] performed the first experiments with lyophilized samples. EPR studies were carried out for samples such as yeast, blood, rabbit organs, germinated digitalis seeds and barley leaves [47]. In the EPR spectrum of whole human blood, partial conversion of hemoglobin to methemoglobin was observed, and physical damage to both molecules was observed by lyophilization. In addition, a free radical signal associated with the breakdown of porphyrin ring structures of hemoglobin was recorded.

Electron paramagnetic resonance (EPR) spectroscopy is the most reliable technique for relationship between reactive oxygen species and disease (or aging), the measurement of biological free radicals and redox states. It has been used in vitro to measure oxygen radicals such as hydroxyl radical and superoxide anion radical in combination with the spin-trapping technique [48]. The measurement of EPR is nondestructive and is unaffected by the turbidity of the sample, so people are interested in using EPR for the in vivo measurement of biological radicals. However, there are difficulties with this. First, steady concentrations of biological radicals are too low to detect directly with EPR spectroscopy during their very short half-life.

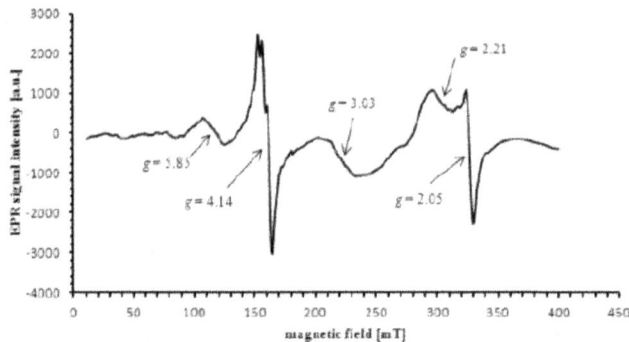

Figure 3. EPR spectrum of whole blood of healthy person contains the signals from Cu^{2+} in ceruloplasmin (g = 2.05), high spin Fe^{3+} in transferrin (g = 4.14), high spin Fe^{3+} in methemoglobin (g = 5.85), low-spin ferriheme complex (g = 2.21) and cytochrome (g = 3.03). Spectrum recorded at 170 K.

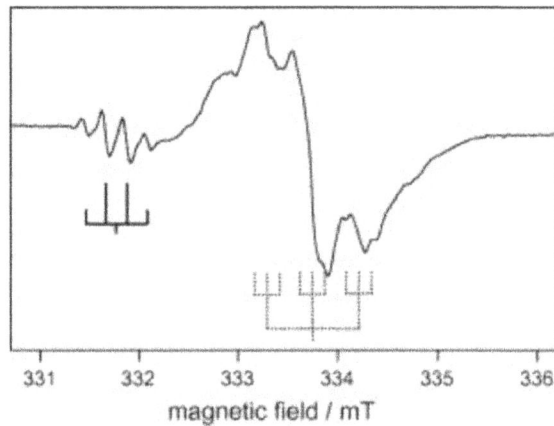

Figure 4. EPR spectrum of the γ-irradiated single crystal of 2-thiothymine.

Second, water in the body of the animal causes dielectric loss of the electromagnetic waves used for EPR measurement [49].

EPR spectra of some biological samples are shown in **Figure 3** [50] and **Figure 4** [51].

7. Conclusion

Free radicals play a role in biological oxidation-reduction reactions, radiation damage, photosynthesis and carcinogenesis. Electron paramagnetic resonance is a very good technique to directly observe free radical intermediates in most of these reactions. In particular, there are many environmental factors that affect human life. It is inevitable that this technique is guiding in discussing the effects of these factors and taking various measures accordingly.

Author details

Betül Çalişkan[1*] and Ali Cengiz Çalişkan[2]

*Address all correspondence to: bcaliska@gmail.com

1 Department of Physics, Faculty of Arts and Science, Pamukkale University, Kinikli, Denizli, Turkey

2 Department of Chemistry, Faculty of Science, Gazi University, Ankara, Turkey

References

[1] Commoner B, Townsend J, Pake GE. Free radicals in biological materials. Nature. 1954;**174**:689-691. DOI: 10.1038/174689a0

[2] McIlwain H. The magnitude of microbial reactions involving vitamin-like compounds. Nature. 1946;**158**(4025):898-902

[3] Blum HF. Light and the melanin pigment of human skin. Annals of the New York Academy of Sciences. 1948;**4**:388-398

[4] Kensler CJ, Dexter SO, Rhoads CP. The inhibition of a diphosphopyridine nucleotide system by split products of dimethylaminoazobenzene. Cancer Research. 1942;**2**:1-10

[5] Lipkin D, Paul DE, Townsend J, Weissman SI. Observations on a class of free radicals derived from aromatic compounds. Science. 1953;**117**(3046):534-535. DOI: 10.1126/science. 117.3046.534

[6] Lyons MJ, Gibson JF, Ingram DJE. Free-radicals produced in cigarette smoke. Nature. 1958;**181**:1003-1004. DOI: 10.1038/1811003a0

[7] Yu LX, Dzikovski BG, Freed JH. A protocol for detecting and scavenging gas-phase free radicals in mainstream cigarette smoke. Journal of Visualized Experiments. 2012; **59**(e3406):1-5. DOI: 10.3791/3406

[8] Steiner PE. The conditional biological activity of the carcinogens in carbon blacks, and its elimination. Cancer Research. 1954;**14**(2):103-110

[9] Krebs HA. In: Sumner JB, Myrback K, editors. The Enzymes. Vol. II. New York: Academic Press; 1951. pp. 1-46

[10] Waters WA. The Chemistry of Free Radicals (Chapter 12). Oxford: Oxford University Press; 1946

[11] Cahill AE, Taube H. One-Electron oxidation of copper Phthalocyanine. Journal of the American Chemical Society. 1951;**73**(6):2847-2851. DOI: 10.1021/ja01150a124

[12] George P, Ingram DJE, Bennett J. One-equivalent intermediates in phthalocyanine and porphin oxidations investigated by paramagnetic resonance. Journal of the American Chemical Society. 1957;**79**(8):1870-1873. DOI: 10.1021/ja01565a027

[13] Gibson JF, Ingram DJE. Location of free electrons in porphin ring complexes. Nature. 1956;**178**:871-872. DOI: 10.1038/178871b0

[14] Gibson JF, Ingram DJE, Nicholls P. Free radical produced in the reaction of metmyoglobin with hydrogen peroxide. Nature. 1958;**181**:1398-1399. DOI: 10.1038/1811398a0

[15] George P, Irvine DH. The reaction between metmyoglobin and hydrogen peroxide. The Biochemical Journal. 1952;**52**(3):511-517

[16] Gibson JF, Ingram DJ, Perutz MF. Orientation of the four haem groups in haemoglobin. Nature. 1956;**178**(4539):906-908. DOI: 10.1038/178906a0

[17] Gibson JF, Ingram DJE. Electron resonance studies of haemoglobin azide and hydroxide derivatives. Nature. 1957;**180**(4575):29-30

[18] Ingram DJE, Kendrew JC. Orientation of the haem group in myoglobin and its relation to the polypeptide chain direction. Nature. 1956;**178**(4539):905-906

[19] Bennett JE, Gibson JF. Electron resonance studies of haemoglobin derivatives. I. Haem plane orientations. Proceedings of the Royal Society A. 1957;**240**(1220):67-82. DOI: 10.1098/rspa.1957.0067

[20] Bennett JE, Gibson JF, Ingram DJ, Haughton TM, Kerkut GA, Munday KA. The investigation of haemoglobin and myoglobin derivatives by electron resonance. Physics in Medicine and Biology. 1957;**1**(4):309-320. DOI: 10.1088/0031-9155/1/4/301

[21] Cohn M, Townsend J. A study of manganous complexes by paramagnetic resonance absorption. Nature. 1954;**173**:1090-1091. DOI: 10.1038/1731090b0

[22] Haber F, Willstätter R. Unpaarigkeit und radikalketten im reaktionsmechanismus organischer und enzymatischer vorgänge. Berichte der Deutschen Chemischen Gesellschaft. 1931;**64**(11):2844-2856. DOI: 10.1002/cber.19310641118

[23] Michaelis L. In: Green DE, editor. Currents in Biochemical Research. New York: Willey Interscience; 1946

[24] Brill AS, Der Hartog H, Legallais V. Fast and sensitive magnetic susceptometer for the study of rapid biochemical reactions. The Review of Scientific Instruments. 1958;**29**(5):383-391. DOI: 10.1063/1.1716203

[25] Pauling L, Coryell CD. The magnetic properties and structure of the hemochromogens and related substances. Proceedings of the National Academy of Sciences of the United States of America. 1936;**22**(3):159-163. DOI: 10.1073/pnas.22.3.159

[26] Adams M, Blois MS Jr, Sands RH. Paramagnetic resonance spectra of some semiquinone free radicals. The Journal of Chemical Physics. 1958;**28**(5):774-776. DOI: 10.1063/1.1744269

[27] Beinert H. Evidence for an intermediate in the oxidation-reduction of flavoproteins. The Journal of Biological Chemistry. 1957;**225**(1):465-478

[28] Commoner B, Lippincott BB, Passonneau JV. Electron-spin resonance studies of free-radical intermediates in oxidation-reduction enzyme systems. Proceedings of the National Academy of Sciences of the United States of America. 1958;**44**(11):1099-1110

[29] Ehrenberg A, Ludwig GD. Free radical formation in reaction between old yellow enzyme and reduced triphosphopyridine nucleotide. Science. 1958;**127**(3307):1177-1178

[30] Bray RC, Malmström BG, Vänngård T. The chemistry of xanthine oxidase. 5. Electron-spin resonance of xanthine oxidase solutions. The Biochemical Journal. 1959;**73**(1):193-197

[31] Malmstrom BG, Vanngard T, Larsson M. An electron-spin-resonance study of the inter-action of manganous ions with enolase and its substrate. Biochimica et Biophysica Acta. 1958;**30**(1):1-5

[32] Malmstrom BG, Mosbach R, Vanngard T. An electron spin resonance study of the state of copper in fungal laccase. Nature. 1959;**183**(4657):321-322

[33] Sands RH, Beinert H. On the function of copper in cytochrome oxidase. Biochemical and Biophysical Research Communications. 1959;**1**(4):175-178. DOI: 10.1016/0006-291X (59)90013-0

[34] Beinert H, Sands RH. On the function of iron in DPNH cytochrome c reductase. Biochem-ical and Biophysical Research Communications. 1959;**1**(4):171-174. DOI: 10.1016/0006-291X (59)90012-9

[35] Hill R, Whittingham CP. Photosynthesis. London: Methuen; 1955

[36] Commoner B, Heise JJ, Townsend J. Light-induced paramagnetism in chloroplasts. Proceedings of the National Academy of Sciences of the United States of America. 1956;**42**(10):710-718

[37] Sogo PB, Pon NG, Calvin M. Photo spin resonance in chlorophyll-containing plant mate-rial. Proceedings of the National Academy of Sciences of the United States of America. 1957;**43**(5):387-393

[38] Tollin G, Calvin M. The luminescence of chlorophyll-containing plant material. Proceed ings of the National Academy of Sciences of the United States of America. 1957;**43**(10): 895-908

[39] Bradley DF, Calvin M. The effect of thioctic acid on the quantum efficiency of the hill reaction in intermittent light. Proceedings of the National Academy of Sciences of the United States of America. 1955;**41**(8):563-571

[40] Arnold W, Sherwood HK. Are chloroplasts semiconductors? Proceedings of the National Academy of Sciences of the United States of America. 1957;**43**(1):105-114

[41] Calvin M, Sogo PB. Primary quantum conversion process in photosynthesis: Electron spin resonance. Science. 1957;**125**(3246):499-500. DOI: 10.1126/science.125.3246.499

[42] Ingram DJE, Symons MCR. Solutions of Sulphur in oleum. Part I. Electron-spin reso-nance of solutions of Sulphur in oleum. Journal of the Chemical Society. 1957:2437-2439. DOI: 10.1039/JR9570002437

[43] Gordy W, Ard WB, Shields H. Microwave spectroscopy of biological substances. I. Paramagnetic resonance in X-irradiated amino acids and proteins. Proceedings of the National Academy of Sciences of the United States of America. 1955;**41**(11):983-996. DOI: 10.1073/pnas.41.11.983

[44] Rexroad HN, Gordy W. Electron-spin resonance studies of radiation damage to certain lipids, hormones, and vitamins. Proceedings of the National Academy of Sciences of the United States of America. 1959;**45**(2):256-269

[45] Shields H, Gordy W. Electron-spin resonance studies of radiation damage to the nucleic acids and their constituents. Proceedings of the National Academy of Sciences of the United States of America. 1959;**45**(2):269-281

[46] Blois MS. Antioxidant determinations by the use of a stable free radical. Nature. 1958;**181**:1199-1200. DOI: 10.1038/1811199a0

[47] Sands RH, Weaver HE, Franken PA. Paramagnetic ions in blood sera. In: Proceedings First Annual Conference of the Biophysical Society. Columbus, Ohio; 1958

[48] Buettner GR. Spin trapping: ESR parameters of spin adducts. Free Radical Biology & Medicine. 1987;**3**(4):259-303. DOI: 10.1016/S0891-5849(87)80033-3

[49] Takeshita K, Ozawa T. Recent progress in in vivo ESR spectroscopy. Journal of Radiation Research. 2004;**45**(3):373-384. DOI: 10.1269/jrr.45.373

[50] Kubiak T, Krzyminiewski R, Dobosz B. EPR study of paramagnetic centers in human blood. Current Topics in Biophysics. 2013;**36**(1):7-13. DOI: 10.2478/ctb-2013-0006

[51] Bešić E, Gomzi V. EPR study of a sulfur-centered π radical in γ-irradiated single crystal of 2-thiothymine. Journal of Molecular Structure. 2008;**876**(1-3):234-239. DOI: 10.1016/j.molstruc.2007.06.033

Chapter 3

Determination of Magnetic Anisotropy by EPR

Andrej Zorko

Additional information is available at the end of the chapter

http://dx.doi.org/10.5772/intechopen.78321

Abstract

Electron paramagnetic resonance (EPR) is a powerful spectroscopic technique, perfectly suited for determining magnetic anisotropy terms in spin Hamiltonians. Although solid foundations of the EPR theory were established by Kubo and Tomita (KT) more than half a century ago, especially in the last couple of decades, we have witnessed a rapid progress in the field due to the occurrence of enhanced computational capabilities. In this chapter, we overview this progress by summarizing the basic concepts of EPR in exchange-coupled systems. The review builds upon the standard KT theory and the exchange narrowing picture, which is however only suitable at high enough temperatures and for systems with dimensionality exceeding one. We also summarize the predictions of more modern approaches, including exact calculations on finite spin clusters, the Oshikawa-Affleck effective-field theory for 1D systems, and the recently developed EPR-moments approach. Many illuminating examples of the applicability of different approaches are also provided.

Keywords: EPR, ESR, EMR, Kubo-Tomita theory, exact diagonalization, Oshikawa-Affleck effective-field theory, EPR moments, exchange-coupled spin systems, magnetic anisotropy, Dzyaloshinskii-Moriya interaction, anisotropic exchange, single-ion anisotropy

1. Introduction

Since the pioneering demonstration of the electron paramagnetic resonance phenomenon in solids and liquids in 1944 by Zavoisky [1–3], EPR has become a well-established and broadly spread spectroscopic technique. Although the main principle of detecting microwave absorption by electronic magnetic moments at a fixed frequency and a sweeping applied magnetic fields has not changes from early days, the method has become one of the most sensitive local probes of magnetism.

The term electron paramagnetic resonance in a narrow sense applies to paramagnetic compounds containing transition-metal or rare-earth elements with incomplete inner shells, hence possessing paramagnetic electron moments. In a broader sense, the general term electron magnetic resonance (EMR) stands for magnetic resonance absorption experiments performed on an ensemble of magnetic moments corresponding to localized or itinerant electrons. In addition to paramagnets, EMR thus also covers absorption phenomena in ordinary metals and magnetically ordered systems, as well as absorption by imperfections in insulators and semiconductors, which may trap electrons or holes. In literature, also the term electron spin resonance (ESR) is often encountered. This is usually reserved for cases when the magnetic moment originates primarily from the spin momentum of the electron, like in iron-group metals where the orbital moment of the electron is usually quenched.

The EPR technique provides superior insight into magnetic properties of a particular sample compared to more conventional bulk magnetic techniques, e.g., bulk-magnetization or magnetic-torque measurements. A particular EPR experiment can provide information that help in characterization of local magnetic and electrostatic environments of a magnetic moment, as well as information about development of magnetic correlations and fluctuations [4–6]. The experiment can also help to determine magnetic coupling with other electronic and nuclear moments, etc. Due to these diverse and detailed information, EPR has earned reputation in various fields of science. Traditionally, it was in the domain of solid-state physics and chemistry, but lately it has become indispensable also in bio-oriented sciences and medical applications. Moreover, it has been recently highlighted for its strength in detecting unconventional magnetic phenomena, such as edge states in topological insulators [7], spinon excitations in spin liquids [8], and spin-nematic states [9].

For a general introduction to EPR the reader is advised to turn to one of many very good EPR monographs and reviews, like the Abragam and Bleaney "Electron Paramagnetic Resonance of Transition Ions" [4], the Pilbrow "Transition Ion Paramagnetic Resonance" [5], or the more recent Weil and Bolton "Electron Paramagnetic Resonance: Elementary Theory and Practical Applications" [6]. The purpose of this chapter is to review a specific problem of EPR in exchange coupled systems. This problem is particularly difficult to treat due to complications induced by the exchange interaction between neighboring moments. These interactions dramatically affect the way the moments respond to the external magnetic fields. In order to model this response properly, the use of modern theoretical concepts and advanced experimental approaches is required. These are review in this chapter.

The outline of the chapter is the following. We will start with a general overview of the Kubo-Tomita EPR theory (Section 2), which will first require the introduction of the spin-Hamiltonian concept. We will pay special attention to the exchange-narrowing limit, which is generally applicable to strongly-exchange-coupled spin systems. Next, a few successful applications of the KT theory will be demonstrated in Section 3. In Section 4, limitations of the KT approach will be summarized. Different approaches that can overcome these limitations and their specific applications will also be given. The concluding Section 5 will summarize this chapter.

2. KT theory of EPR in exchange-coupled systems

Dense magnetic insulators, i.e., systems that do not conduct electric current and where magnetic moments are localized at well-defined crystallographic sites (usually occupied by transition metals or rare earths), represent one of the major fields of research in condensed matter, where EPR is particularly powerful [10]. In this chapter, we shall focus on systems that are strongly exchange coupled, i.e., where magnetic moments communicate, and highlight particular information that EPR can provide in such cases.

EPR measures the absorption of microwaves by electrons, i.e., atomic magnetic moments, therefore, it provides a direct insight to the atomic magnetism. This is unlike some other local-probe techniques, such as nuclear magnetic resonance [11, 12] or muon spectroscopy [13] that can only provide indirect information about electron degrees of freedom. However, as we shall see below, this advantage of EPR at the same time turns out to be a drawback, since knowledge of four-spin correlations functions is required to accurately describe the EPR response of exchange-coupled magnetic moments at an arbitrary temperature. On the other hand, for indirect techniques, like NMR, two-spin correction functions suffice. This makes EPR an elaborate technique and prevents a routine analysis of the EPR spectra of exchange-coupled systems.

The beginnings of the EPR theory in exchange-couples magnetic systems go back to the seminal work by Kubo and Tomita (KT) entitled "General Theory of Magnetic Resonance Absorption" [14]. Although it rests on a perturbation approach and is therefore not exact, the KT theory still represents solid foundations in modern times. The EPR theory has seen some progress later on, especially in recent years with the advent of enhanced computational facilities. Within this chapter, we shall make a general overview of the KT theory and its successors that were developed for cases where the KT theory is not valid.

2.1. Spin Hamiltonian

We start the body of this review with introducing the concept of the spin Hamiltonian. In this framework the total Hamiltonian of a particular system with all degrees of freedom that are present, i.e., electron orbital, electron spin, nuclear, lattice, etc., is projected onto the spin space of the electrons. In an external magnetic field, the spin Hamiltonian comprises of the following terms [6]:

$$H = H_Z + H_{hf} + H_{ex} + H'. \tag{1}$$

Here, $H_Z = \mu_B \vec{B_0} \cdot \underline{g} \cdot \vec{S}$ is the Zeeman interaction of the electronic spin $\vec{S}$ with the applied magnetic field $\vec{B_0}$ (μ_0 denotes the Bohr magneton, $\underline{g}$ is the g tensor), H_{hf} is the electron-nuclear hyperfine coupling interaction,

$$H_{ex} = \sum_{i,\, j>i} J_{ij} \vec{S_i} \cdot \vec{S_j} \tag{2}$$

is the exchange Hamiltonian summing terms between electron spins at sites i and j coupled by an isotropic exchange interaction J_{ij}, and H' represents magnetic anisotropy. The latter,

$$H' = H_{dd} + H_{zfs} + H_{AE} + H_{DM},$$ (3)

includes the dipolar term between electronic spins H_{dd}, the zero-field splitting term H_{zfs}, which reflects a combined effect of the electrostatic crystal field and spin-orbit coupling on the energy levels in spin space, the symmetric anisotropic exchange (AE) term

$$H_{AE} = \sum_{i,j>i} \vec{S}_i \cdot \underline{\delta} \cdot \vec{S}_j,$$ (4)

where $\underline{\delta}$ is the symmetric part of the anisotropic exchange tensor, and the antisymmetric anisotropic exchange term

$$H_{DM} = \sum_{i,j>i} \vec{d}_{i,j} \cdot \vec{S}_i \times \vec{S}_j,$$ (5)

known as the Dzyaloshinskii-Moriya (DM) interaction ($\vec{d}$ is the DM vector) [15, 16]. We note that the dipolar term is important in diluted magnetic systems, but is usually negligible in dense magnetic insulators. The zero-field splitting term may be important for spins $S > 1/2$ and has, in the lowest order in spin, the following form

$$H_{zfs} = D\left(S_z^2 - S(S+1)/3\right) + E\left(S_x^2 - S_y^2\right).$$ (6)

The exchange anisotropy is a relativistic effect due to the spin-orbit coupling. In transition metals, the Dzyaloshinskii-Moriya interaction is usually the dominant exchange anisotropy term. The reason is that it originates from the first-order perturbation in the spin-orbit coupling, while the symmetric anisotropic exchange results only from the second-order perturbation theory [15, 16]. Consequently, the DM term is proportional to $(\Delta g/g)J$, while the symmetric AE term is proportional to $(\Delta g/g)^2 J$, where the g-shift Δg from the free electron value of 2.0023 measures the amount of the orbital momentum in the ground crystal-field state due to mixing of higher crystal-field states. In copper-based magnets, for example, one typically finds $\Delta g/g \approx 0.15$ [4, 5].

2.2. EPR spectrum

In the high-temperature limit, where thermal energy is larger than the Zeeman energy splitting (in the conventional X-band at 9.5 GHz the Zeeman spitting corresponds to the temperature of 0.45 K), the EPR absorption spectrum is determined in the linear-response theory by thermal-averaged (denoted by $\langle \ldots \rangle$) fluctuations of the total transverse spin operator $\vec{S} = \sum_i \vec{S}_i$, as [14].

$$I(\omega) \propto \omega \chi''(\omega) \propto \frac{\omega}{T} \int\limits_{-\infty}^{\infty} \langle S^+(t)S^-(0)\rangle e^{-i\omega t} dt, \tag{7}$$

where the spin ladder operators are given by $S^{\pm} = S^x \pm iS^y$ and $\chi''(\omega)$ represents the imaginary part of the uniform dynamical susceptibility. In the case when the Zeeman interaction is dominant, one can separate the Hamiltonian $H_0 = H_{ex} + H_Z$ from the other, perturbing terms H'. Rewriting $\chi''(\omega)$ in the interaction representation, which is given by the transformation $\tilde{S}(t) = e^{-iH_0t/\hbar}S(t)e^{iH_0t/\hbar}$, then yields

$$\chi''(\omega) \propto \int\limits_{-\infty}^{\infty} \left(\langle \tilde{S}^+(t)S^-(0)\rangle e^{-i(\omega-\omega_0)t} + \langle \tilde{S}^-(t)S^+(0)\rangle e^{-i(\omega+\omega_0)t} \right) dt. \tag{8}$$

Eq. (8) reveals an interesting result that the resonant absorption is peaked at the Larmor frequency $\pm\omega_0 = g\mu_B B_0/\hbar$, where $\hbar$ is the reduced Planck constant. Moreover, in the case of no anisotropy, there is no time dependence of the spin correlation functions in the interaction representation (Eq. (8)), therefore the EPR spectrum simply consists of two δ-functions. The time dependence of the correlation functions in Eq. (8), which is due to magnetic anisotropy H', is thus solely responsible for finite line widths of the EPR spectra and their shifts from the Larmor frequency. This is an essential results, as it demonstrates that magnetic anisotropy is directly reflected in the shape of the EPR line spectrum, unlike in all other techniques capable of detecting the anisotropy, e.g., inelastic neutron scattering, where the signal is a combined effect of multiple factors. Usually the EPR line width is small compared to the Larmor frequency and one can neglect the contribution peaked at the negative frequency $-\omega_0$.

According to the KT theory, the EPR spectrum can be expressed as the Fourier transform of the relaxation function $\varphi(t) = \langle \tilde{S}^+(t)S^-(0)\rangle/\langle \tilde{S}^+(0)S^-(0)\rangle$,

$$I(\omega) \propto \int\limits_{-\infty}^{\infty} \varphi(t)e^{-i(\omega-\omega_0)t} dt. \tag{9}$$

Thus, spin correlations embedded into the relaxation function determine the EPR spectrum. The calculation of the relaxation function is however nontrivial. Therefore, approximation schemes are required. For Markovian random processes the relaxation function is approximated by [14]

$$\varphi(0) = \exp\left(-\int\limits_0^t (t-\tau)\psi(\tau)d\tau \right). \tag{10}$$

Here, the spin correlation function is defined as

$$\psi(\tau) = \frac{\langle [\tilde{H}'(0), S^+(0)] [S^-(0), \tilde{H}'(0)] \rangle}{\hbar^2 \langle S^+(0)S^-(0)\rangle}, \tag{11}$$

where $[A, B]$ stands for the commutator between operators A and B. Within the KT theory a Gaussian decay of the spin correlation function is postulated,

$$\psi(0) = \psi(0)e^{-\tau^2/2\tau_c^2}, \tag{12}$$

where the characteristic spin correlation time is determined by the dominant isotropic exchange J, $\tau_c \approx h/J$.

2.3. Exchange narrowing

Let us inspect two limiting cases of the correlation time with respect to the typical EPR time scale given by the Larmor frequency. For slow decay of correlations ($\omega_0\tau_c \gg 1$), i.e., in the quasi-static limit, $\psi(t)$ in Eq. (10) can be replaced by its zero-time value, which is proportional to the second moment of the absorption line

$$M_2 = \hbar^2\psi(0) = \frac{\left\langle \left[H'(0), S^+(0)\right]\left[S^-(0), H'(0)\right]\right\rangle}{\langle S^+(0)S^-(0)\rangle}. \tag{13}$$

This procedure yields a Gaussian relaxation function $\varphi(t)$ and, according to Eq. (9), also a Gaussian shaped EPR spectrum, with the width $\Delta B_G \propto \sqrt{M_2}$.

The fast decay limit ($\omega_0\tau_c \ll 1$) gives a completely different result. Here, the integral in Eq. (10) is approximated by

$$\int_0^t (t - \tau)\psi(\tau)d\tau = \psi(0)\left(t \int_0^{t\to\infty} e^{-\tau^2/2\tau_c^2}d\tau - \int_0^{t\to\infty} \tau e^{-\tau^2/2\tau_c^2}d\tau \right) \approx \sqrt{\frac{\pi}{2}}\frac{M_2}{\hbar^2}\tau_c t, \tag{14}$$

which leads to an exponential decay of the relaxation function $\varphi(t)$. Consequently, the EPR spectrum has a Lorentzian shape. Its line width is $\Delta B_L \propto \tau_c M_2$. As $\tau_c \approx h/J$, this is known as the exchange-narrowing limit [17, 18], where the EPR broadening, which is given by magnetic anisotropy yielding finite M_2, is opposed by the isotropic exchange interaction causing narrowing of the EPR line. The spin correlation time $\tau_c \propto h\sqrt{M_2/M_4}$ is approximated by the second moment (Eq. (13)) and the fourth moment of the absorption line

$$M_4 = \frac{\left\langle \left[H - H_Z, \left[H', S^+(0)\right]\right]\left[H - H_Z, \left[H', S^-(0)\right]\right]\right\rangle}{\langle S^+(0)S^-(0)\rangle}, \tag{15}$$

which yields the full width at half maximum (FWHM) of the Lorentzian EPR line

$$\Delta B = \frac{C}{g\mu_B}\sqrt{\frac{M_2^3}{M_4}}. \tag{16}$$

The exchange-narrowing limit is typically applicable to real exchange-coupled system, except in cases of small couplings and high Larmor frequencies. We recall again that in the most widespread X-band EPR experiment ($\omega_0 = 2\pi \times 9.5$ GHz) a typical temperature scale is 0.45 K. The exchange narrowing is straightforwardly confirmed in an EPR experiment by the Lorentzian line shape of the spectrum. However, strictly speaking, the experimental line shape is never truly Lorentzian, because the moments of the latter diverge, while the EPR moments, given by the commutators, such as those in Eq. (13) and Eq. (15), are always finite. In systems with strong isotropic exchange compared to magnetic anisotropy, deviations from the Lorentzian shape occur only in far wings of the EPR spectrum and are often not even observable. An approximate line shape that is a product of the Lorentzian and a broad Gaussian $\propto \exp\left(-(B - B_0)^2/2B_{ex}^2\right)$, with the exchange field $B_{ex} = k_B\sqrt{M_2/M_4}/g\mu_B$ [19], is then justified. This yields the constant $C = \sqrt{2\pi}$ in Eq. (16). The EPR line width is thus a fingerprint of magnetic anisotropy (Eq. (3)) present in a given exchange-coupled spin system, as the latter yields finite EPR moments (Eq. (13) and Eq. (15)).

3. Applications of the KT theory

Applications of the KT theory to experiments are numerous. Here, we will highlight a few cases from recent literature, where determination of the magnetic anisotropy turned out to be crucial for understanding the magnetic ground state. All examples concern magnetically frustrated spin lattices in 2D, where short-range spin interactions are incompatible with the underlying spin lattices, effectively suppressing long-range spin ordering and leading to unconventional states of matter. In such cases magnetic anisotropy, even if only being a small perturbation to the dominant isotropic exchange interaction, can tip the balance in favor of one or another competing ground state.

3.1. Kagome lattice

The first example is the 2D spin lattice in herbertsmithite, $ZnCu_3(OH)_6Cl_2$ [20], a compound that has earned the reputation of being the best experimental realization of a quantum kagome antiferromagnet (QKA) of corner-sharing triangles (**Figure 1**), where the geometrical frustration is the most severe [21]. Numerous theoretical studies that proposed various different ground states over the last two decades, now seem to have converged on a gapped quantum spin liquid (QSL) – a state that is disordered, yet highly entangled [21]. Experimental signatures of such a state have also been lately advocated, although the bulk of experiments on this and the majority of other known QKA representatives actually speaks in favor of a gapless QSL. This discrepancy may well be related to perturbations beyond the isotropic Heisenberg exchange model on the kagome lattice, such as magnetic anisotropy.

The magnetic anisotropy of herbertsmithite was successfully determined by EPR in Ref. [22]. Based on relatively small g-shifts (of the order of 15%, as typical for Cu^{2+} ions [4, 5]), it was argued that the antisymmetric DM interaction (Eq. (5)) dominates the magnetic anisotropy in this compound. The DM vector pattern (**Figure 1**), which is determined by the symmetry of the kagome lattice, then according to Eq. (16) predicts the following angular dependence of the EPR line width [22]

$$\Delta B(\theta) = \sqrt{2\pi} \frac{k_B}{2g(\theta)\mu_B J} \sqrt{\frac{\left(2d_z^2 + 3d_p^2 + \left(2d_z^2 - d_p^2\right)\cos^2\theta\right)^3}{16d_z^2 + 78d_p^2 + \left(16d_z^2 - 26d_p^2\right)\cos^2\theta}}, \quad (17)$$

where θ represents the polar angle between the normal to kagome planes and the applied magnetic field direction, while d_p and d_z are the in-plane and the out-of-plane components of the DM interaction. This expression is valid only in the infinite-temperature limit, therefore the authors applied it to fit the room-temperature EPR spectrum of herbertsmithite (**Figure 1**), where the EPR line width was shown to saturate to a constant value [22]. Thus the minute in-plane DM component $d_p/J \sim 0.01(3)$ and the dominant out-of-plane DM component $d_z/J \sim 0.08(1)$ could be determined. The magnitude of the extracted DM interaction agrees with another estimate $0.06 < d_z/J < 0.10$, later obtained from NMR measurements [23]. Importantly, this places the system to a QSL part of a phase diagram, however, quite close to a quantum critical point determined by the out-of-plane DM component, which according to theory should occur at $d_z/J \simeq 0.10$ [24]. This point separates the spin-liquid phase from a Néel ordered phase at larger DM values. A further in-depth EPR study has revealed that the establishment of the spin-liquid state in herbertsmithite induces macroscopic symmetry reduction of the crystal lattice [25].

In contrast to herbertsmithite, in another QKA representative, vesignieite, $BaCu_3V_2O_8(OH)_2$, a long-range magnetic order was observed [26], which could be due to the fact that this systems is positioned in the ordered part of the above-mentioned phase diagram. In order to

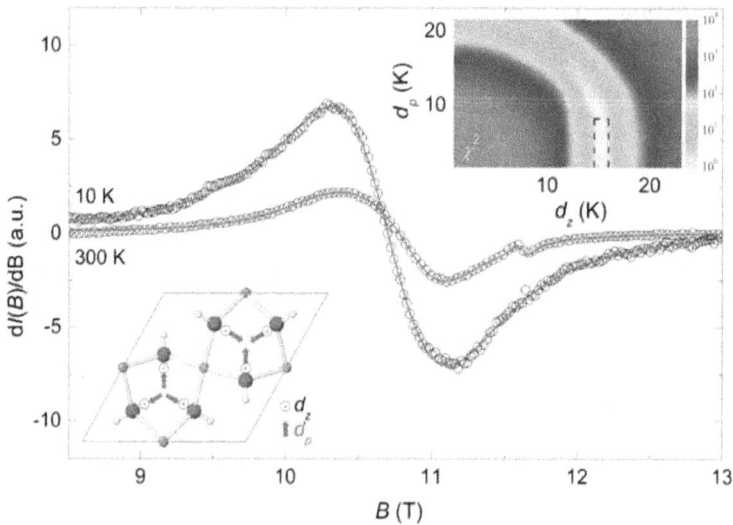

Figure 1. The EPR spectra of $ZnCu_3(OH)_6Cl_2$ at two different temperatures (symbols) and corresponding fits with a model based on the EPR line-width anisotropy given by Eq. (17). The lower inset shows the corresponding kagome lattice of Cu^{2+} $S = 1/2$ spins (orange) and the DM vector pattern. The upper inset shows the quality of the fit (reduced χ^2), where the dashed rectangle highlights the best fitting parameters. (Adapted from ref. [22].)

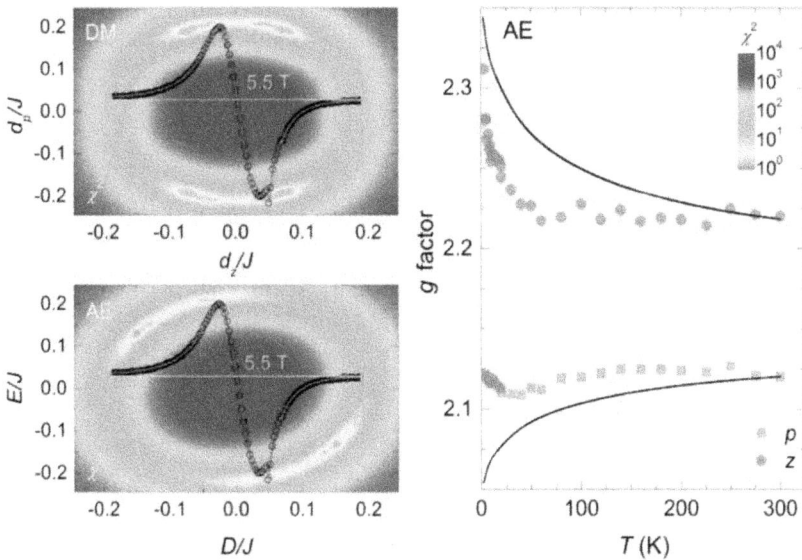

Figure 2. The 300-K EPR spectrum of $BaCu_3V_2O_8(OH)_2$ (symbols) fit with (top left) the DM model of Eq. (17) and (bottom left) the AE model [27] and the corresponding quality of the fits reflected in the reduced χ^2 in the parameter space of each model. (Right) the temperature dependence of the g factor (symbols) and the prediction of the AE model. (Adapted from ref. [27].)

verify this conjecture, the same EPR analysis (**Figure 2**) as the one presented above for herbertsmithite was performed in Ref. [27]. The derived DM components are somewhat different from those in herbertsmithite, as the in-plane component dominates in vesignieite, $d_p/J \sim 0.19(2)$ and $d_z/J \sim 0.07(3)$. Alternatively, the EPR line shape could be modeled also with the symmetric AE model (**Figure 2**). However, the extracted symmetric anisotropy parameters that, contrary to the DM interaction, are responsible also for temperature-dependent EPR shifts, significantly overestimated the measured shifts (**Figure 2**). Therefore, the conclusion was reached, that the DM interaction also dominates in vesignieite. Furthermore, it was argued that the condition $d_p > d_z$ could profoundly affect the quantum critical point because the in-plane DM component disfavors spin structures from the ground-state manifold of the isotropic J and should be much more efficient in suppressing quantum fluctuations than the out-of-plane DM component [27]. This could explain why magnetic ordering in vesignieite occurs at surprisingly high temperature for a frustrated system, $T_N/J \sim 0.17$ [26], despite d_z/J being very similar to the ratio in herbertsmithite.

3.2. Triangular lattice

A regular triangular lattice of edge-sharing triangles is another example of a highly frustrated spin lattice in 2D. Contrary to the kagome lattice, where each spin in surrounded by four nearest neighbors, on the triangular lattice there are six such neighbors, which reduces the

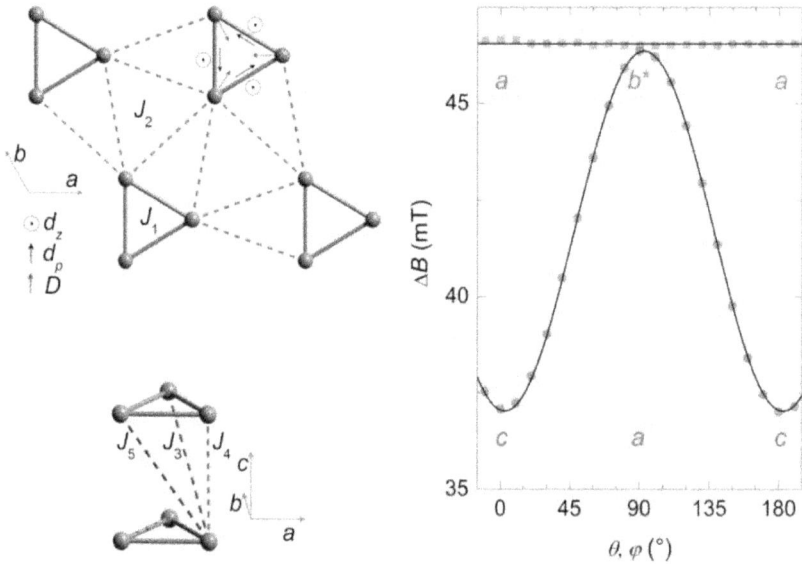

Figure 3. (Left) The 2D triangular arrangement of the Fe^{3+} S = 5/2 spins in $Ba_3NbFe_3Si_2O_{14}$ and the corresponding isotropic exchange interactions $J_1 - J_5$. The basic motif of anisotropic DM and AE interactions is also shown. (Right) The angular dependence of the EPR line width at 500 K (symbols) and the fits (lines) with the model of Eq. (18). (Adapted from ref. [29].)

amount of frustration. Consequently, the triangular lattice exhibits a magnetically ordered ground state, which is, however, much more complex than on ordinary bi-partite spin lattices.

A slightly more complicated triangular lattice is realized in Fe-langasite, $Ba_3NbFe_3Si_2O_{14}$ [28]. Here the Fe^{3+} (S = 5/2) spins reside on vertices of equilateral triangles arranged into a 2D triangular lattice (**Figure 3**). Quite interestingly, the magnetically ordered ground state below T_N = 26 K is doubly chiral, as the same 120° spin configuration on each triangle is helically modulated from plane to plane [28].

To identify the anisotropy term that is responsible for such chirality of the magnetic ground state, an EPR study was again conducted [29]. The room-temperature EPR signal was found to exhibit a pronounced angular dependence of the EPR line width and line position. The former could be related either to zero-field-splitting anisotropy (Eq. (6)) or DM exchange anisotropy (Eq. (5)), with the anisotropy patterns as shown in **Figure 3**. The two models could not be distinguished solely based on the EPR response of the system. However, a combined study of the EPR spectra and antiferromagnetic resonance (AFMR) modes observed below T_N suggested the DM interaction as the dominant source of anisotropy and thus to be responsible for the observed chiral behavior of Fe-langasite. The out-of-plane DM component $d_z/J \sim 0.004$ and the in-plane component $d_p/d_z = 2.6$ were estimated from the combined fits of the EPR and AFMR data. For the EPR line width in accordance with Eq. (16), the DM anisotropy yielded the EPR line width of the form [29]

$$\Delta B(\theta) = \sqrt{2\pi} \frac{k_B}{2g(\theta)\mu_B} \sqrt{\frac{105\left(5d_p^2 + 6d_z^2 + \left(d_p^2 - 2d_z^2\right)\cos 2\theta\right)^3}{32\left(35J_{DM}^2 d_p^2 + 6J_{DM}'^2 d_z^2 + \left(2J_{DM}'^2 d_z^2 - 7J_{DM}^2 d_p^2\right)\cos 2\theta\right)}}, \tag{18}$$

which was fit to the experimentally determined line-width anisotropy at 500 K (**Figure 3**). Here the constants $J_{DM}^2 = 3J_1^2 + 2J_2^2 + J_3^2 + J_4^2 + J_5^2$ and $J_{DM}'^2 = 18J_1^2 + 14J_2^2 + 7J_3^2 + 7J_4^2 + 7J_5^2$ are defined by the five strongest exchange interaction depicted in **Figure 3**.

A later study combining EPR, AFMR and inelastic neutron scattering refined the anisotropy model in Fe-langasite and showed that actually both the DM anisotropy ($d_z/J \sim 0.033$, $d_p/d_z = 2.6$), and the zero-field-splitting anisotropy ($D/J \sim 0.052$) are of very similar size [30].

4. Pitfalls of the KT theory and alternative approaches

Although the above examples nicely demonstrate the value of the KT theory, this theory should be applied to each particular case with caution, because it is limited in several aspects. Firstly, the KT approach does not take into account a possible hidden symmetry of the DM interaction (Section 4.1) and diffusional decay of spin correlations in low dimensional spin systems (Section 4.2). Secondly, the EPR moments (Eq. (13) and Eq. (15)) implicitly employ four-spin correlation functions, which can be explicitly evaluated only in the infinite-temperature limit, where spin correlations between neighboring sites are negligible. On the other hand, the analysis of the EPR line width at temperatures of the order of the dominant exchange coupling J and below requires different approaches, like the Oshikawa-Afflect effective-field-theory (Section 4.3). Lastly, one should keep in mind that the KT theory is perturbative, therefore the cases of large (or even dominant) magnetic anisotropy should be treated with different approaches (Section 4.4).

4.1. Reducibility of the DM interaction

It was found theoretically that the DM interaction may in some cases possess a hidden symmetry [31], in the sense that it can be effectively transformed into a term with the symmetry of the anisotropic exchange and with reduced magnitude of d^2/J, by applying a nonuniform spin rotation [32]. Consequently, the exchange narrowing KT theory becomes inadequate for describing the effect of the DM interaction on the ESR line width. However, this is true only for certain spin lattices and certain components of the DM interaction [33]. The components that can be eliminated in the first order in d are those that sum up to zero within any closed loop on a spin lattice; for example, for the kagome lattice, the in-plane DM component D_p is reducible, while the out-of-plane component D_z is irreducible. The KT theory remains applicable for the irreducible components of the DM interaction.

4.2. Spin diffusion

In low-dimensional magnetic systems it may happen that the Gaussian approximation of the decay of the spin correlation function in Eq. (12) is not justified due to a diffusional contribution to the decay. This dictates slower time dependence of the form [34].

$$\psi(\tau) \propto \tau^{-D/2}, \tag{19}$$

where D represents the dimensionality of the spin system. For $D \leq 2$ this leads to a divergent integral in Eq. (14), which in reality leads to broadening of the EPR spectra and changes their shape from the Lorentzian shape [34].

When the secular part of the anisotropy Hamiltonian (Eq. (3)), i.e., the part commuting with the Hamiltonian H_0, dominates the anisotropy in one-dimensional systems, the relaxation function is given by $\varphi(t) = \exp\left(-(\Gamma t)^{3/2}\right)$, where $\Gamma = \left(4M_2/3\hbar^2\right)^{2/3}\tau_c^{1/3}$ [34]. The Fourier transform in Eq. (9) then yields an absorption spectrum decaying somewhere in-between the Lorentzian and the Gaussian line shape (**Figure 4**). The line width of the spectrum is of the order of Γ. On the other hand, there exists no universal picture for two dimensions. Nevertheless, deviations of the experimentally observed EPR spectra from the Lorentzian shape in 2D were observed in the past and successfully ascribed to the presence of spin diffusion [35]. Quite generally, the spin-diffusion effect in two dimensions is usually much less pronounced than in one dimension.

Finally, we note that the diffusional decay of the electronic spin correlation functions is often not detectable by EPR at all, even in low dimensional systems. Although these systems may be

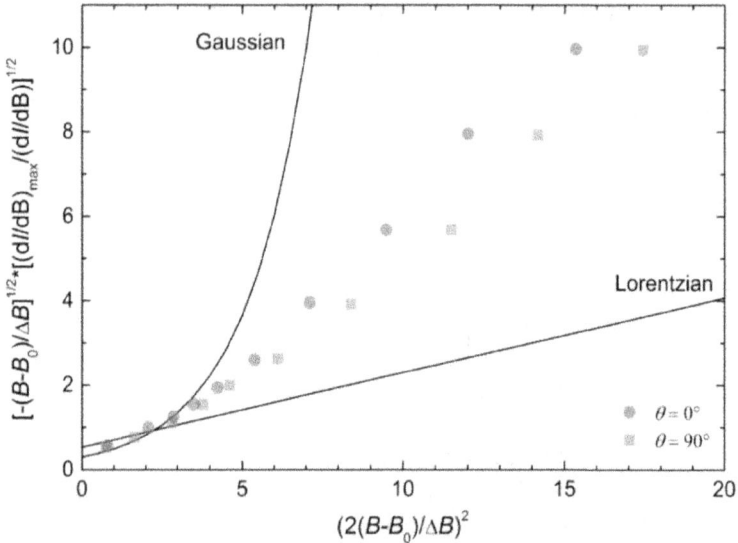

Figure 4. Analysis of the line shape in the one-dimensional spin system $(CH_3)_4NMnCl_3$ (TMMC) for two different directions of the magnetic field. (Adapted from ref. [34].)

characterized as being low dimensional due to the dominant exchange interaction along a chain or within a plane, also inter-chain/inter-layer exchange couplings can still be large compared to the magnetic anisotropy terms regulating the linewidth of the EPR absorption spectra. In such cases the decay of spin correlations is effectively taking place in three dimensions and the spin-diffusion problem is absent.

4.3. Exact calculations on finite clusters

The postulate of the Gaussian decay of the spin correlation function in the KT theory (Eq. (12)) has no theoretical background and is not necessarily valid, as explained in Section 4.1. However, this assumption is not needed at all if the EPR line shape is calculated from the basics, i.e., from Eq. (7). This can be done only on finite clusters of spins. Such a limitation then requires an extrapolation to the thermodynamic limit if these calculations are to be applied to macroscopic samples.

Exact calculations of the EPR line shape on finite clusters were performed by El Shawish et al. [36] for certain 1D and 2D spin lattices. For a spin chain, the results showed a noticeable transformation of the decay of the spin correlations from the Gaussian shape at early times to a much slower decay of diffusional characteristics at longer times. The resulting line broadening and the deviation from the Lorentzian line shape were, however, later shown to be effectively short-cut by inter-chain exchange [37].

The situation is very different in 2D, e.g., for the kagome spin lattice. Namely, the finite-cluster calculations revealed that, at least for the irreducible DM component d_z the line width indeed scales with d_z^2/J [36], as predicted by the KT theory. Although no clear signature of the diffusional decay of spin correlations was observed, an interpolation to the spin-diffusional assumption still caused a moderate increase of the line width and a slight deviation from the Lorentzian line shape. For herbertsmithite, such an assumption would then slightly decrease the amplitude of the DM vector compared to the above-presented results based on the KT approach, namely to $0.04 \leq d_z/J \leq 0.08$ [36].

We note that the finite-cluster approach is severely limited, as the extrapolation to the thermodynamic limit, which is usually of interest in experiments, is highly nontrivial and depends on a particular spin lattice [36]. However, since the results are exact, this approach may still be very interesting for small systems, such as molecular magnets. An interesting prediction of a double-peak EPR spectrum was also given (**Figure 5**). The spectrum should thus strongly differ from the usual Lorentzian line shape, which still awaits experimental confirmation.

4.4. Oshikawa-Affleck theory

Exact calculations of the second and fourth moments of the EPR absorption spectra (Eq. (13) and Eq. (15)) are possible within the KT framework for infinite lattices, but only in the limit of infinite temperature. In this case, static spin correlations of the products of spin operators acting on different lattice sites can be neglected. In general, in Eq. (13) and Eq. (15), one is dealing with the computation of four-spin correlation functions since the magnetic anisotropy

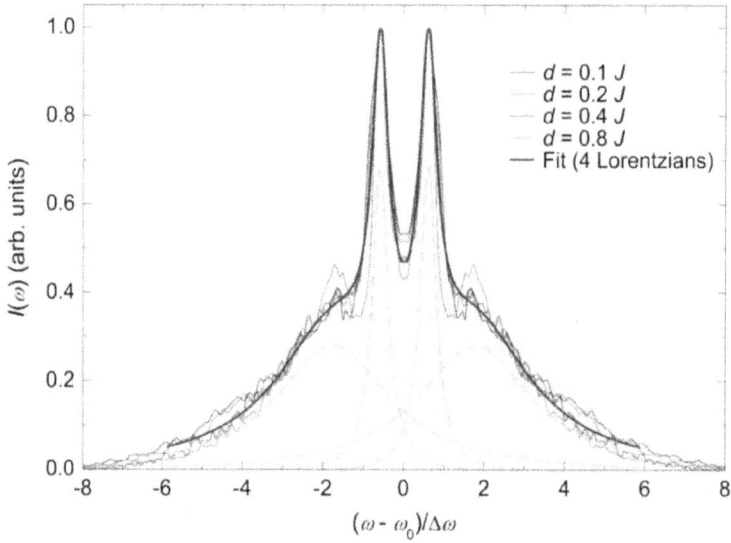

Figure 5. The EPR line shape of a finite 16-spin chain for different values of the staggered DM interaction d. The curves are rescaled with the half width $\Delta\omega$. (Adapted from ref. [36].)

Hamiltonian is quadratic in spin operators. Therefore, special schemes of disentangling the four-spin correlation functions into products of two-spin correlation functions need to be applied [14, 19]. Further complications emerge at finite temperatures, i.e., at $T \sim J$, when spin correlations between adjacent spin sites become important.

The problem of how finite temperatures (finite spin correlations) affect the EPR line width is treated within the Oshikawa-Afflect effective-field-theory approach that is applicable to spin chains [38, 39]. The spin diffusion picture, which predicts a non-Lorentzian line shape in 1D, does not apply to the OA theory. In contrast to the KT theory, this approach works well at intermediate and low temperatures, $T_N \ll T \ll J$, where, in general, all classical theories break down due to many-body correlation effects. The lower limit is given by the Néel temperature of 3D spin ordering, where 3D critical spin correlations develop. The AO theory allows to differentiate between the symmetric-exchange-anisotropy broadening and the antisymmetric DM broadening, as different scalings with temperature and magnetic field are predicted. The AE contribution scales like [38–40]

$$\Delta B_{AE}(T) = \varepsilon \frac{2k_B(\delta/J)^2}{g\mu_B\pi^3} T, \tag{20}$$

where the constant $\varepsilon = 2$ applies for the direction of the external magnetic field along the anisotropy axis and $\varepsilon = 1$ for the perpendicular directions. This contribution does not depend on the magnitude of the applied field and scales linearly with temperature. The DM contribution to the EPR line width is characterized by the staggered field $h_s = c_s B_0$, where the staggered field coefficient c_s originates from the DM interaction and/or from a staggered g factor. This broadening is of the form

$$\Delta B_{DM}(T, B_0) = 0.69 g \mu_B \frac{k_B J}{(k_B T)^2} h_s^2 \sqrt{\ln\left(\frac{J}{T}\right)}. \tag{21}$$

The temperature dependence of the DM broadening is inverse to the AE broadening, as the former decreases with increasing temperature while the latter increases. Moreover, while the AE broadening effect is independent of the applied field, the DM broadening increases with the square of the applied field.

If both the AE and the DM term are of similar magnitude in a particular system, one can expect to observe both EPR broadening mechanisms simultaneously. Such is, for instance, the case in the $CuSe_2O_5$ spin-chain compound [40]. There, simultaneous modeling of the angular, temperature, and frequency-dependent EPR line width with the OA theory (the sum of contributions in Eq. (20) and Eq. (21)) allowed Herak et al. to extract both the AE and the DM anisotropy constants [40]. The simultaneous fits of the AO theory to multiple experimental datasets are presented in **Figure 6**.

At the end, it should be stressed that the OA approach still relies on the perturbation theory (in magnetic anisotropy). So, cases, where the anisotropy is of the order of the isotropic exchange interactions or larger are untreatable within this theory.

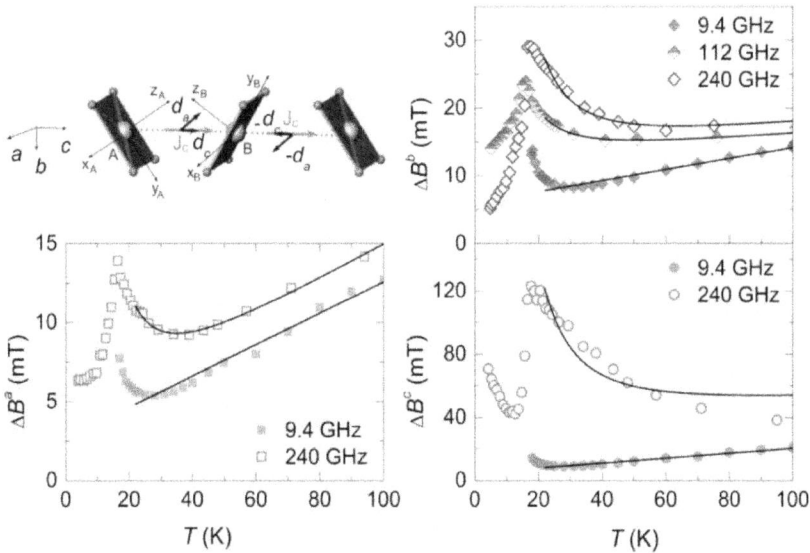

Figure 6. (top left) A 1D chains of Cu^{2+} S = 1/2 spins (orange) in $CuSe_2O_5$. Other panels show the temperature dependence of the EPR line width in three crystallographic directions at different frequencies. The solid lines are fits to the OA theory of the data (symbols) corrected for high-temperature phonon-induced broadening. (Adopted from ref. [40].)

4.5. EPR moments

The EPR-moments approach [41] described in this section is more direct, i.e., non-perturbative. Within this approach the line width (and line shift) in the "frequency domain," where the frequency is varied in a fixed Zeeman field, can be calculated for an arbitrary strength of magnetic anisotropy. Moreover, exact calculations at any temperature are possible for spin chains. In general, the EPR line width is given by the four lowest shifted moments

$$
m_n^\omega = J^{-n} \int_{-\infty}^{\infty} (\omega - h)^n \chi''(\omega - h) d\omega, \tag{22}
$$

where $h = g\mu_B B_0/\hbar$, as [41]

$$
\Delta\omega = J^2 \frac{Jm_3^\omega + hm_2^\omega}{Jm_2^\omega + hm_1^\omega} - \left(J \frac{Jm_2^\omega + hm_1^\omega}{Jm_1^\omega + hm_0^\omega} \right)^2 . \tag{23}
$$

The moments in the frequency domain (Eq. (22)) represent static correlations that can be calculated in the case of 1D spin chains to arbitrary precision for any temperature and applied field [41]. The agreement of this approach with fully numerical calculation for finite chain Hamiltonians is shown in **Figure 7**.

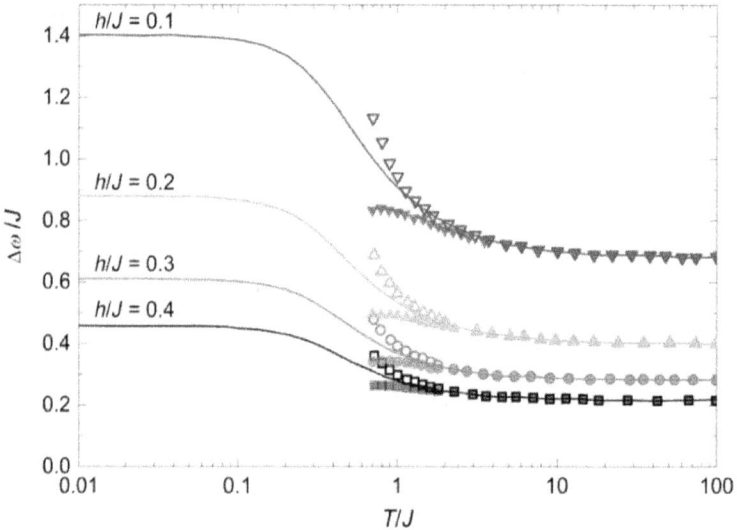

Figure 7. The temperature dependence of the EPR line width in the frequency domain of a spin chain predicted by the EPR moments approach (Eq. (23)) for the AE anisotropy $\delta = 0.1\ J$ at various fields $h = g\mu_B B_0/k_B$ (lines). The symbols represent numerical calculations on finite chains with the length of $N = 16$ spins (full symbols) and $N = 24$ spins (open symbols). (Adopted from ref. [41].)

In a typical EPR experiment, however, the frequency is kept constant and the magnetic field is swept. It turns out that the calculation of the shifted moments in the field domain,

$$m_n^h = J^{-n} \int\limits_{-\infty}^{\infty} (\omega - h)^n \chi''(\omega - h) \mathrm{d}h, \tag{24}$$

requires the knowledge of infinitely many moments in the frequency domain. Therefore, the experimental line width cannot be calculated exactly at arbitrary temperature and field [40].

We should stress that the fact the EPR spectrum is measured in a field-sweet experiment is actually neglected in almost all theoretical treatments. Furthermore, a complication that arises when applying the EPR-moments approach to an experiment is that "long tails" of the EPR line may considerably contribute to the moments, while these are usually not properly accounted for by the experimentally determined FWHM due to noise [42]. Therefore a cutoff of high-frequency tails is necessary, as it was recently demonstrated for the case of the quasi-one-dimensional magnet $Cu(py)_2Br_2$ [42].

5. Conclusions

This chapter reviews the development of the treatment of the EPR absorption line in strongly exchange-coupled spin systems. The starting point is the Kubo Tomita general theory of magnetic resonance absorption, which demonstrates how the line width can be approximated by two lowest even moments of the EPR line, M_2 and M_4. We note that the knowledge of all the moments, $M_n = \int_{-\infty}^{\infty} \omega^n I(\omega) \mathrm{d}\omega$, is equivalent to the knowledge of all the derivatives of a particular absorption line and, therefore, exactly determines the line shape. A particularly enlightening result of the KT theory is the phenomenon of exchange narrowing, according to which the EPR line width scales with the square of the magnetic anisotropy and is inversely proportional to the isotropic exchange interaction.

The KT approach was successfully applied to various spin lattices in the past, including the geometrically frustrated kagome and triangular lattices, which are exemplified here. However, when the theory is applied to a particular system special attentions needs to be made a) to a possible reducibility of the asymmetric Dzyaloshinskii-Moriya exchange anisotropy, b) to the diffusional decay of spin correlations, which may occur in low-dimensional spin systems, c) to finite correlations among spins at different sites, which typically develop below the temperature of the order of the dominant isotropic exchange, and d) to the size of the magnetic anisotropy, which is only treated as a perturbation in the KT theory. All these drawbacks of the KT theory can be overcome, at least in special cases. In this review, special approaches that were developed in this vein have been summarized. These include a) exact calculations of the EPR line on finite clusters, the Oshikawa-Affleck effective-field theory for 1D spin systems, and the recently developed EPR-moments approach. For each approach a representative example has been provided in this review.

Acknowledgements

The author acknowledges the financial support of the Slovenian Research Agency under the program No. P1-0125.

Conflict of interest

The author declares no conflict of interests.

Author details

Andrej Zorko

Address all correspondence to: andrej.zorko@ijs.si

Jožef Stefan Institute, Ljubljana, Slovenia

References

[1] Zavoisky EK. Solutions and metals [thesis]. In: Absorption in Orthogonal and Parallel Fields for Salts. Kazan: Kazan University; 1944

[2] Zavoisky EK. Journal of Physics (USSR). 1945;**9**:211

[3] Zavoisky EK. Journal of Physics (USSR). 1945;**9**:245

[4] Abragam A, Bleaney B. Electron Paramagnetic Resonance of Transition Ions. Oxford: Clarendon Press; 1970. 911 pp

[5] Pilbrow JR. Transition Ion Electron Paramagnetic Resonance. Oxford: Clarendon Press; 1990. 717 pp

[6] Weil JA, Bolton JR. Electron Paramagnetic Resonance: Elementary Theory and Practical Applications. 2nd ed. Hoboken: John Wiley & Sons; 2007. 664 pp. DOI: 10.1002/0470084987

[7] Yao Y, Sato M, Nakamura T, Furukawa N, Oshikawa M. Theory of electron spin resonance in one-dimensional topological insulators with spin-orbit couplings: Detection of edge states. Physical Review B. 2017;**96**:205424-1-205424-10. DOI: 10.1103/PhysRevB.96.205424

[8] Luo ZX, Lake E, Mei JW, Starykh OA. Spinon magnetic resonance of quantum spin liquids. Physical Review Letters. 2018;**120**:037204-1-037204-6. DOI: 10.1103/PhysRevLett.120.037204

[9] Furuya SC, Momoi T. Electron spin resonance for the detection of long-range spin nematic order. Physical Review B. 2018;**97**:104411-1-104411-18. DOI: 10.1103/PhysRevB.97.104411

[10] Bencini A, Gatteschi D. EPR of Exchange Coupled Systems. Berlin: Springer-Verlag; 1990. 287 pp. DOI: 10.1007/978-3-642-74599-7

[11] Abragam A. The Principles of Nuclear Magnetism. Oxford: Oxford University Press; 1961. 599 pp

[12] Slichter CP. Principles of Magnetic Resonance. 3rd ed. Berlin: Springer-Verlag; 1996. 655 pp. DOI: 10.1007/978-3-662-09441-9

[13] Yaouanc A, De Réotier PD. Muon Spin Rotation, Relaxation, and Resonance: Applications to Condensed Matter. Oxford: Oxford University Press; 2011. 486 pp

[14] Kubo R, Tomita K. A general theory of magnetic resonance absorption. Journal of the Physical Society of Japan. 1954;9:888-919. DOI: 10.1143/JPSJ.9.888

[15] Dzyaloshinsky I. A thermodynamic theory of weak ferromagnetism of antiferromagnetics. Journal of Physics and Chemistry of Solids. 1958;4:241-255. DOI: 10.1016/0022-3697(58)90076-3

[16] Moriya T. Anisotropic superexchange interaction and weak ferromagnetism. Physics Review. 1960;120:91-98. DOI: 10.1103/PhysRev.120.91

[17] Van Vleck JH. The dipolar broadening of magnetic resonance lines in crystals. Physics Review. 1948;74:1168-1183. DOI: 10.1103/PhysRev.74.1168

[18] Anderson PW, Weiss PR. Exchange narrowing in paramagnetic resonance. Reviews of Modern Physics. 1953;25:269-276. DOI: 10.1103/RevModPhys.25.269

[19] Castner Jr. TG, Seehra MS. Antisymmetric exchange and exchange-narrowed electron-paramagnetic-resonance linewidths. Physical Review B. 1971;4:38-45. DOI: 10.1103/PhysRevB.4.38

[20] Shores MP, Nytko EA, Bartlett BM, Nocera DG. A structurally perfect S = 1/2 Kagomé Antiferromagnet. Journal of the American Chemical Society. 2005;127:13462-13463. DOI: 10.1021/ja053891p

[21] Norman MR. Colloquium: Herbertsmithite and the search for the quantum spin liquid. Reviews of Modern Physics. 2016;88:041002-1-041002-14. DOI: 10.1103/RevModPhys.88.041002

[22] Zorko A, Nellutla S, van Tol J, Brunel LC, Bert F, Duc F, Trombe JC, De Vries MA, Harrison A, Mendels P. Dzyaloshinsky-Moriya anisotropy in the spin-1/2 kagome compound $ZnCu_3(OH)_6Cl_{12}$. Physical Review Letters. 2008;101:026405-1-026405-4. DOI: 10.1103/Phys RevLett.101.026405

[23] Rousochatzakis I, Manmana SR, Läuchli AM, Normand B, Mila F. Dzyaloshinskii–Moriya anisotropy and nonmagnetic impurities in the S = 1/2 kagome system $ZnCu_3(OH)_6Cl_2$. Physical Review B. 2009;79:214415-1-214415-11. DOI: 10.1103/PhysRevB.79.214415

[24] Cépas O, Fong CM, Leung PW, Lhuillier C. Quantum phase transition induced by Dzyaloshinskii–Moriya interactions in the kagome antiferromagnet. Physical Review B. 2008;78:140405-1-140405-4. DOI: 10.1103/PhysRevB.78.140405

[25] Zorko A, Herak M, Gomilšek M, van Tol J, Velázquez M, Khuntia P, Bert F, Mendels P. Symmetry reduction in the quantum Kagome Antiferromagnet Herbertsmithite. Physical Review Letters. 2017;**118**:017202-1-017202-16. DOI: 10.1103/PhysRevLett.118.017202

[26] Yoshida M, Okamoto Y, Takigawa M, Hiroi Z. Magnetic order in the spin-1/2 kagome antiferromagnet vesignieite. Journal of the Physical Society of Japan. 2012;**82**:013702-1-013702-4. DOI: 10.7566/JPSJ.82.013702

[27] Zorko A, Bert F, Ozarowski A, van Tol J, Boldrin D, Wills AS, Mendels P. Dzyaloshinsky–Moriya interaction in vesignieite: A route to freezing in a quantum kagome antiferromagnet. Physical Review B. 2013;**88**:144419-1-144419-7. DOI: 10.1103/PhysRevB.88.144419

[28] Marty K, Simonet V, Ressouche E, Ballou R, Lejay P, Bordet P. Single domain magnetic Helicity and triangular Chirality in structurally Enantiopure $Ba_3NbFe_3Si_2O_{14}$. Physical Review Letters. 2008;**101**:247201-1-247201-4. DOI: 10.1103/PhysRevLett.101.247201

[29] Zorko A, Pregelj M, Potočnik A, Van Tol J, Ozarowski A, Simonet V, Lejay P, Petit S, Ballou R. Role of antisymmetric exchange in selecting magnetic chirality in $Ba_3NbFe_3Si_2O_{14}$. Physical Review Letters. 2011;**107**:257203-1-257203-5. DOI: 10.1103/PhysRevLett.107.257203

[30] Chaix L, Ballou R, Cano A, Petit S, de Brion S, Ollivier J, Regnault LP, Ressouche E, Constable E, Colin CV, Zorko A, Scagnoli V, Balay J, Lejay P, Simonet V. Helical bunching and symmetry lowering inducing multiferroicity in Fe langasites. Physical Review B. 2016;**93**:214419-1-214419-5. DOI: 10.1103/PhysRevB.93.214419

[31] Shekhtman L, Entin-Wohlman O, Aharony A. Moriya's anisotropic superexchange interaction, frustration, and Dzyaloshinsky's weak ferromagnetism. Physical Review Letters. 1992;**69**:836-839. DOI: 10.1103/PhysRevLett.69.836

[32] Choukroun J, Richard JL, Stepanov A. High-temperature electron paramagnetic resonance in magnets with the Dzyaloshinskii–Moriya interaction. Physical Review Letters. 2001;**87**:127207-1-127207-4. DOI: 10.1103/PhysRevLett.87.127207

[33] Cheng YF, Cépas O, Leung PW, Ziman T. Magnon dispersion and anisotropies in $SrCu_2$$(BO_3)_2$. Physical Review B. 2007;**75**:144422-1-144422-10. DOI: 10.1103/PhysRevB.75.144422

[34] Dietz RE, Merritt FR, Dingle R, Hone D, Silbernagel BG, Richards PM. Exchange narrowing in one-dimensional systems. Physical Review Letters. 1971;**26**:1186-1188. DOI: 10.1103/PhysRevLett.26.1186

[35] Richards PM, Salamon MB. Exchange narrowing of electron spin resonance in a two-dimensional system. Physical Review B. 1974;**9**:32-45. DOI: 10.1103/PhysRevB.9.32

[36] El Shawish S, Cépas O, Miyashita S. Electron spin resonance in $S = 1/2$ antiferromagnets at high temperature. Physical Review B. 2010;**81**:224421-1-224421-9. DOI: 10.1103/PhysRevB.81.224421

[37] Furuya SC, Sato M. Electron spin resonance in quasi-one-dimensional quantum antiferromagnets: Relevance of weak interchain interactions. Journal of the Physical Society of Japan. 2015;**84**:033704-1-033704-5. DOI: 10.7566/JPSJ.84.033704

[38] Oshikawa M, Affleck I. Low-temperature electron spin resonance theory for half-integer spin antiferromagnetic chains. Physical Review Letters. 1999;**82**:5136-5139. DOI: 10.1103/PhysRevLett.82.5136

[39] Oshikawa M, Affleck I. Electron spin resonance in S = 1/2 antiferromagnetic chains. Physical Review B. 2002;**65**:134410-1-134410-28. DOI: 10.1103/PhysRevB.65.134410

[40] Herak M, Zorko A, Arčon D, Potočnik A, Klanjšek M, van Tol J, Ozarowski A, Berger H. Symmetric and antisymmetric exchange anisotropies in quasi-one-dimensional $CuSe_2O_5$ as revealed by ESR. Physical Review B. 2011;**84**:184436-1-184436-8. DOI: 10.1103/PhysRevB.84.184436

[41] Brockmann M, Göhmann F, Karbach M, Klümper A, Weiße A. Theory of microwave absorption by the spin-1/2 Heisenberg-Ising magnet. Physical Review Letters. 2011;**107**:017202-1-017202-5. DOI: 10.1103/PhysRevLett.107.017202

[42] Zeisner J, Brockmann M, Zimmermann S, Weiße A, Thede M, Ressouche E, Povarov KY, Zheludev A, Klümper A, Büchner B, Kataev V, Göhmann F. Anisotropic magnetic interactions and spin dynamics in the spin-chain compound cu(py)$_2$Br$_2$: An experimental and theoretical study. Physical Review B. 2017;**96**:024429-1-024429-24. DOI: 10.1103/PhysRevB.96.024429

Chapter 4

EPR Methods Applied on Food Analysis

Chryssoula Drouza, Smaragda Spanou and
Anastasios D. Keramidas

Additional information is available at the end of the chapter

http://dx.doi.org/10.5772/intechopen.79844

Abstract

An overview of the different methodologies developed so far for the investigation of paramagnetic species in foods is presented. Electron paramagnetic resonance spectroscopy (EPR), also known as electron spin resonance spectroscopy (ESR), is the primary technique toward the development of methods for the exploration of EPR-sensitive species, such as free radicals, reactive oxygen species (ROS), nitrogen reactive species (NRS), and C-centered radicals and metal ions. These methods aim for: (a) quantification of radical species, (b) exploration of redox chemical reaction mechanisms in foods, (c) assessment of the antioxidant capacity of food, and (d) food quality, stability, and food shelf life. For these purposes, different radical initiations and detections have been used in foods depending on both the chemistry of the target system and the kind of information required, listed in: the induction of radicals by (a) microwave, UV, or γ-radiation; (b) heating; (c) addition of metals; and (d) use of oxidants.

Keywords: EPR, free radicals, food, antioxidants, spin traps, time-dependent EPR

1. Introduction

In the last few years, the applications of the magnetic resonance techniques, particularly nuclear magnetic resonance (NMR) and electron paramagnetic resonance (EPR), in food chemistry have enormously increased [1–5].

EPR spectroscopy is a sensitive and versatile technique for analyzing molecules that contain unpaired electrons, such as paramagnetic metal ions and organic radicals. The formation of organic radicals in foods is an indication of food degradation occurring mainly due to oxidation reactions. Metal ions present in foods are able to catalyze oxidation of the food components by activating O_2 to produce reactive oxygen species (ROS). In addition to the analysis of the paramagnetic species in foods, EPR can be used for the evaluation of the food stability and shelf-life. In order to perform such studies, acceleration of the radical production and degradation in food is needed. Several methods have been applied for the production of radicals in foods, including irradiation with microwave, UV, or γ-radiation, heating, and addition of oxidants. Stable organic radicals, such as tyrosyl and semiquinone radicals, can be detected directly by EPR. However, for the detection of transient radicals, spin traps are employed in order to be measured by EPR spectroscopy. The life of the short-lived radicals can also be extended by rapid freezing of the samples after their generation. In addition, time-resolved EPR can be used for the detection of short-lived radicals. Valuable information is acquired for the mechanisms involved in these reactions by measuring the EPR signal *vs* time.

The main objective of this chapter is the discussion of methods for food analysis by cw X-band EPR, including the observation of endogenous unpaired electronic spin species and the initiation and detection of free radicals in foods.

2. Endogenous unpaired electronic spin species in foods

2.1. Metal ions in food

Foods contain metal ions originated either from the raw starting materials or from contamination with metals from metallic containers or from contamination with metals during food processing [6–9]. EPR spectroscopy is particularly sensitive in detection of Fe^{III}, Mn^{II}, and Cu^{II} metal ions, which can be found in food materials, because of their relative long relaxation times. Fe^{III} gives at X-band EPR a singlet at ~160 mT, Mn^{II} a six-line hyperfine pattern due to the coupling of the unpaired electrons with ^{55}Mn nucleus (spin $I = 5/2$) at 300–350 mT, while Cu^{II} gives quartet hyperfine splitting after coupling with ^{59}Cu nucleus (spin $I = 3/2$) for the isotropic spectra at room temperature at 250–320 mT. The axial anisotropic EPR spectra of Cu^{II} nucleus consist of four peaks for the magnetic field aligned along the z axis and one peak for the magnetic field aligned along xy plane. One example was provided by Drew et al. who employed cw X-band EPR to explore the origin of the metal ions in Scotch whiskies [7].

The EPR spectrum of a frozen whiskey, depicted in **Figure 1**, shows the presence of all three metal ions.

The EPR spectra of Mn^{II} is of particular interest because Mn^{II} is present at almost all the foods of plant origin [10]. The signal of the frozen solutions of the symmetric $[Mn^{II}(H_2O)_6]^{2+}$ consists of six narrow lines with additional small peaks between the six main components due to forbidden transitions. However, the EPR signal of Mn^{II} is significantly different from $[Mn^{II}(H_2O)_6]^{2+}$ when Mn^{II} is coordinated to small ligands or large biomolecules mainly because of changes in zero field splitting (ZFS) parameters [11, 12]. These EPR data can be obtained from the simulations of the experimental spectra and they can be used for investigating the coordination environment around Mn^{II} in foods. However, foods are complicated biosystems and metal ions might interact with several molecules creating around them various environments [13] of different symmetry.

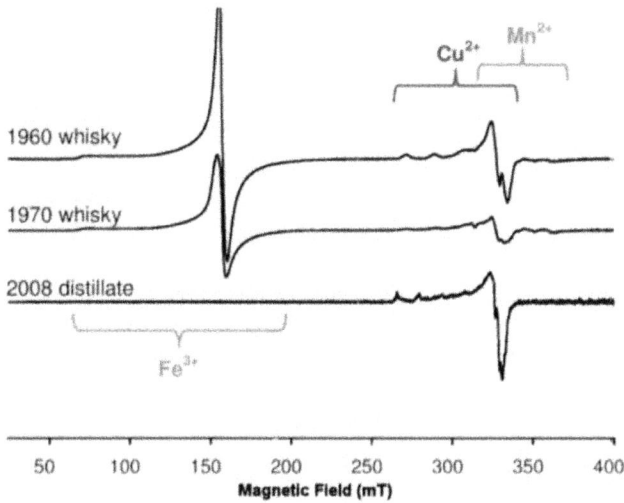

Figure 1. Cw X-band EPR spectra of a 2008 distillate and as-bottled aged whiskies from 1960 to 1970. After the permission of Prof. SC Drew.

Thus, the Mn^{II} EPR signal is complicated and fitting of the signal by considering one Mn^{II} species is not possible in most of the cases. In order to analyze the multicomponent EPR signals, researchers combine EPR and separation techniques and analyze the EPR signals of simpler-paramagnetic fractions [14].

Trials to fit the Mn^{II} EPR signal of two Cypriot wines using Easyspin 5.2.8 [15] (**Figure 2**) did not result in a perfect match with the experimental spectra revealing multiple Mn^{II} species in the wines.

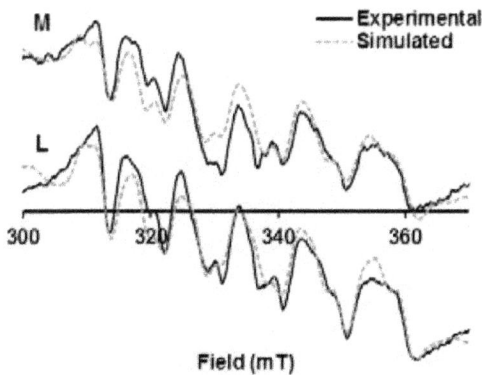

Figure 2. Experimental (black continues lines) and simulated (red dashed lines) cw X-band EPR spectra of two Cypriot wines from the grapes varieties Lefkada (L) and Maratheftiko (M) at 110 K. For the simulations were used the following parameters: (L) $g = 1.999$, $A = 258$ MHz, $D = 530$ MHz, and $E = 192$ MHz; (M) $g = 1.999$, $A = 257$ MHz, $D = 564$ MHz, and $E = 210$ MHz.

These EPR spectra features of the metal ions, which are originated from the various environments occurring for metal ions in foods, might be used for the food classification such as geographical or botanical discrimination. An example of the use of Mn^{II} X-band EPR spectroscopy for the discrimination of Cypriot wines from various grape varieties is shown in **Figure 3** (unpublished results). In addition to the characteristic shape of the spectrum, the quantity of Mn^{II} in each wine can be measured from the double-integrated spectra in the presence of standard [14, 16] information that can be additionally used as a variable for the wine discrimination.

The Mn^{II} cw X-band EPR spectra are also useful for analyzing the degradation of the food [10, 17]. An example of the alternation of the Mn^{II} signal in the wines up to exposure to air is shown in **Figure 4**. After the exposure, a new signal is appeared at $g = 2.000$ and $A \sim 185$ MHz. Such signals have been assigned to multinuclear manganese clusters of higher oxidation states than Mn^{II} as previously reported for studies in solutions of model Mn^{II} compounds after their exposure to O_2 [18, 19]; therefore, similar clusters might be formed also in wines.

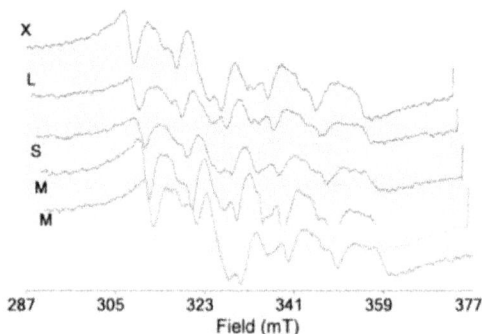

Figure 3. Cw X-band EPR spectra of various Cypriot wines from the grape varieties Xynisteri (X), Lefkada (L), Shiraz (S), and Maratheftiko (M) at 110 K.

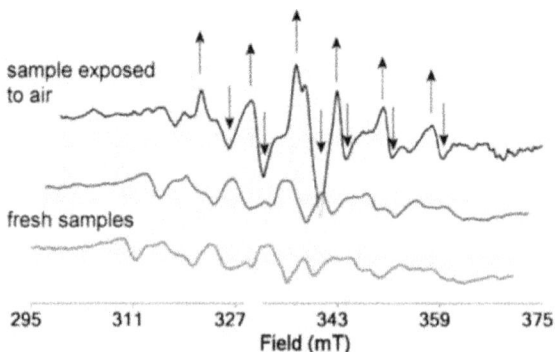

Figure 4. Cw X-band EPR spectra of two fresh samples and one sample exposed to atmospheric oxygen for 1 day of the Cypriot wine from the grape variety Maratheftiko (M) at 110 K.

The presence of free ions, such as Fe^{III} and Cu^{II}, might accelerate degradation of foods, through Fenton reactions, leading to undesirable taste, color, or food spoilage [20–26]. Sometimes the removal of excessive free ions from foods is required in order to preserve their quality [8]. Metal chelators have found to inhibit the oxidation and increase the stability of model wines [27]. On the other hand, addition of metal ions in foods emerges reactive radical species that can be detected by EPR and used further for food characterization.

2.2. Organic radicals

In addition to metallic radicals, foods might contain persistent organic radicals formed by the exposure of food in atmospheric oxygen or the food preparation processes. Metal ions might play an important catalytic role in the formation of organic radicals. For example, although X-band EPR spectrum of fresh tea leaves gives at $g = 2.000$ only the sextet of Mn^{II}, the ground tea from tea bags gives a sharp peak due to the stable semiquinone radical, in addition to the Mn^{II} peak (**Figure 5**).

An extensive EPR study of dry tea leaves from various origins has shown that except the semiquinone radicals, stable carbohydrate radical can also be detected [28]. The same study showed that the type of radical is depended on the content of flavan-3-ols in tea. The teas owned the highest content of flavan-3-ols (unfermented teas) form carbohydrate radicals, whereas fermented teas have high quantities of semiquinone radicals.

Troup et al. have investigated the organic radicals formed in roasted coffee beans and the brewed coffee solutions by EPR spectroscopy [14]. They have assigned the radicals to high-molecular-weight phenolic compounds present in the coffee brew and melanoidin compounds generated in the course of the Maillard reaction from reducing sugars and amino acids.

Phenolics are also the compounds which form radicals in red wines [29]. In addition, stable radicals were detected directly in the extracts of carrot root, celery stalk, cress shoots, cucumber, parsley, and cabbage leaf appeared upon maceration. The EPR signal is a double peak in the EPR spectrum, attributed to the monodehydroascorbyl radical formed in the aqueous

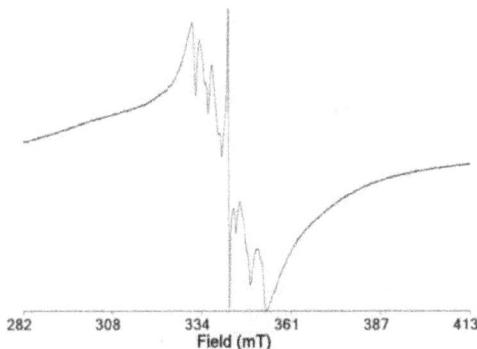

Figure 5. Cw X-band EPR spectra of ground tea from tea bags at room temperature.

solution. A wide single peak overlays the above signals in some samples and is attributed to the stressed biotic or abiotic conditions [30].

In general, fresh foods, protected from the oxidation, do not form organic radicals. However, such radicals might be induced and used for the characterization of food shelf-stability.

3. Induction and monitoring of radicals in foods

3.1. Methods for induction of radicals

Several methods have been used for the induction of free radicals in foods, including irradiation with UV, microwaves, or γ-radiation, heating, addition of ozone, metal ions, or other oxidants. The EPR signal of stable radicals formed in food could be monitored directly, whereas unstable radicals can be measured indirectly with the addition of spin traps.

The use of EPR spectroscopy to monitor radicals in γ-radiated foods is a common practice which is very well documented in the literature [31–39]. The most of the studies were focused on consumer safety due to the use of this method in some countries for food product sterilization.

Microwave irradiation also causes formation of radicals in foods which can be monitored by EPR spectroscopy [40]. X-band EPR studies of the effect of microwave radiation on rice flour and rice starch [41–43] have shown the formation of tyrosyl and semiquinone radicals, after food irradiation, localized in the starch and the protein fraction of rice flour. These radicals exist in the native rice flour; however, their intensity increases exponentially by increasing microwave power and radiation time. The authors have proposed that transition metal redox process might be associated with the formation of the radicals [42, 43]. On the other hand, the rate of radical generation in flour starch is not related to the microwave power and irradiation time but increases rapidly at about $100°C$ [41].

UV-irradiation is a very popular technique for the generation of radicals measured by EPR [44–46]. Foods are directly irradiated with UV-light [47–49] or after the addition of a photosensitive radical initiator in foods [50, 51]. The radicals, produced from UV-irradiation, usually are trapped by spin traps before being measured by EPR. However, there are examples of direct measurement of stable radicals formed in food. For example, UV-irradiation of grains resulted in the formation of reactive oxygen species and stable semiquinone and phenoxyl radicals [49]. In addition to the formation of organic radicals, the Mn^{II} and the Fe^{III} EPR signals alternate, pointing to a disturbance of the biomolecules' structures.

The thermal stability of foods, in particular, edible oils, is a property associated with the storage life of food staff explored through various spectroscopic methods and rancimat analysis [52–57]. The thermal process of foods generates radicals that can be detected by EPR spectroscopy. An example of heating-induced radical formation is the coffee beans roasting with formed radicals to be monitored in real time [14, 58, 59]. Goodman et al. have shown that the organic radicals produced from the heating of coffee beans are dependent on the variety of the bean, but the experimental data were not enough to support an explanation. In addition, they noticed that the quantity of radicals is higher at the presence of O_2, and the oxidation rate of beans is considerably higher during the cooling process [58]. The radicals produced from the heating of edible oils are trapped with radical traps such as N-tert-butyl-α-phenylnitrone (PBN). Monitoring the signal of the PBN spin adducts by EPR consists a promising method for the determination of the lipid oxidation lag phase but not suitable for the lag phase of hydroperoxides and thus oil shelf-life [60]. The formation of free radicals in edible oils is catalyzed by unsaturated lipids, and in this autoxidation mechanism, there is a direct involvement of β-carotene and chlorophyll [61]. The EPR spectra of the heated oils showed also the formation of α-tocopheryl radical, suggesting that the α-tocopheryl radical might be used as an alternative marker for studying the oxidation state of edible oils [61, 62]. The EPR spectra of edible oils heated at 180 °C in contact with metals suggested that iron and aluminum do not significantly affect the oils. On the other hand, heating the oil with copper resulted in the dissolution of large quantities of Cu^{II} in the oil promoting the decomposition of primary oxidation products, while increasing the buildup of secondary oxidation products [63].

Ozone is a nonthermal technology with promising application in food processing. It is primarily used as a disinfectant and antimicrobial agent for food safety applications and for food preservation [64–66]. However, processing of foods with ozone results in the formation of radicals that can be detected with EPR [67, 68]. The ozonation of grains was found to be safe for the consumers; however, the application of ozone directly on food products containing crushed grains, for instance, meal, might pose a threat to consumers.

The initiation of radicals with addition of metal ions or with the addition of metal ions with H_2O_2 (Fenton-like reagents) is also a usual strategy for the characterization of foods. The formation of radicals with the Fenton reagents is based in the reactions (1) and (2).

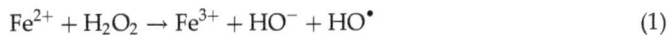

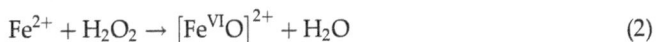

$$Fe^{2+} + H_2O_2 \rightarrow Fe^{3+} + HO^- + HO^\bullet \tag{1}$$

$$Fe^{2+} + H_2O_2 \rightarrow \left[Fe^{VI}O\right]^{2+} + H_2O \tag{2}$$

However, in addition to Fenton reagent, other reagents [69], reacting like the Fenton reagent, such as Co^{II}/H_2O_2, Cu^I/H_2O_2 [70], and $K_2S_2O_8$ [71], might be used. Usually, the radicals formed from the reaction with the Fenton reagents are trapped by spin traps and monitored by various spectroscopies including EPR. This methodology has been applied on several types of foods including plant extracts [72], strawberry fruit [73], sugar and other molecules found in foods [74], edible oils [48, 75], tea [76], wines [27], etc. Investigation of the reactivity of Fe^{II} complexes with quinolinic acid as Fenton reagent has shown that Fe(II)-Quin produces more hydroxyl radicals and is more stable than Fe(II) alone [72]. In addition, metal ions being in the form of salts are insoluble in lipids; thus, in order to be used as radical initiators in lipids, they require their solubility to be increased by the addition of emulsifiers [77–79]. Recently, Drouza et al. have synthesized lipophilic metal complexes soluble in oils that initiate radicals in the presence of oxygen [3], whereas α-tocopherol is used as a marker for the investigation of the olive oils' stability.

3.2. Addition of radicals

A common use of EPR spectroscopy is the addition of reactive organic radicals, usually DPPH[•], galvanoxyl radical, ABTS[+•], TEMPO, TEMPOL, or Fremy's salt for the determination of the antioxidant activity of foods [80–84]. The EPR signal is reduced after the addition of radicals in oil because of the reduction of the radicals from the antioxidant food components, and the antioxidant activity can be calculated from Eq. (3) or more complicate mathematical equations [85–89].

$$Inhibition\ activity\% = (A_0 - A)/A_0 \times 100 \tag{3}$$

where A_0 and A are the double integrals of the signal of the control and the sample after the addition of the antioxidant, respectively.

Stable radicals can also be added as probes. The EPR signal of the radical is dependent on the environment around the radical, thus structural information can be acquired. The radical probes could be organic [90–94] or inorganic [13]. The X-band EPR spectra of aqueous solutions containing extracts of green or black tea and Cu^{II} showed the formation of six complexes, probably of Cu^{II} with amino acids. The interactions of Cu^{II} with teas are pH dependent. At high pH, the Cu^{II} ions form complexes with polyphenols [13].

3.3. Lipophilic metal initiators

Although metal ions have been used as insoluble salts to induce free radicals in edible oil samples, a novel approach has been presented by the utilization of lipophilic metal complexes as radical initiators for the oxidation of lipids in olive oils, targeting the activation of α-tocopheryl radical naturally contained in edible oils [3].

The new metal initiators consist the V^V and V^{IV} complexes, **1** and **2** (**Figure 6**), containing a lipophilic tail enabling them to perfectly dissolve in the oil matrix. This has been presented as an advantage of the new method because it allows the retaining of the chemical environment neighboring the polar phenols as it is in the bulk pure oil. Thus, phenols are allowed to participate in the free radical interplay between the redox species unaffected by any phase

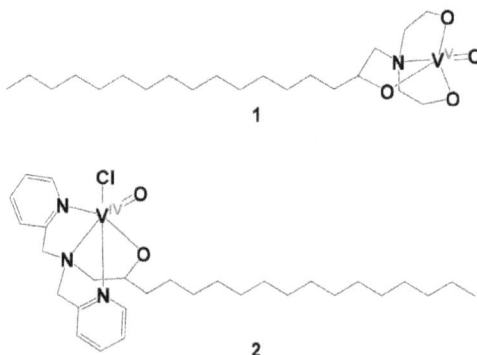

Figure 6. Vanadium (IV/V) complexes **1** and **2**.

change discontinuation as it occurred in the case of the emulsions. In this method, the evolution of the phenol scavenging activity is recorded versus time revealing information for all the time framework of the food exposure to radicals (**Figures 7** and **8**).

The particular metal ion, vanadium, was selected because it participates in redox reactions, producing radicals and stabilizing semiquinone radicals [95–97], and activate molecular dioxygen [98, 99]. Cw X-band variable temperature (VT)-EPR spectroscopy reveals strong interactions between complex **2** and phenols suggesting that such interactions in the presence of O_2 might promote the initiation of the radicals.

The effect of the polar phenols naturally contained in the edible oils on the dioxygen activation and the free radical production was explored by a key experiment based on the monitoring of the intensity of the EPR α-tocopheryl signal in the presence and/or the absence of the polar phenols. The subtraction of the polar phenols resulted in (i) the reduction of maximum intensity of the EPR signal of α-tocopheryl radical and (ii) the decrease of the time needed for the occurrence of maximum intensity, tm, for the same edible oil. This new method has been applied for evaluating the age of olive oil or the storage period associated with the amounts of the polar phenols, which are decomposed by the increase of the storage time, using the

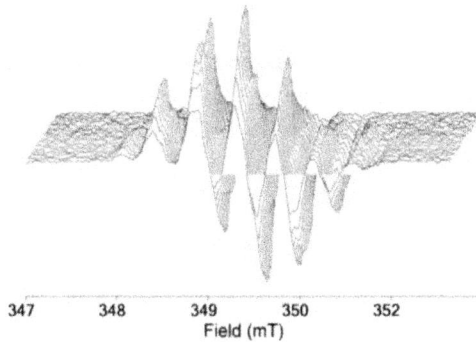

Figure 7. X-band EPR spectrum of virgin olive oil (0.500 g) *vs* time after addition of **1** (100 µL, 7.00 mM) at RT. The time period between two adjacent spectra is 6.5 min.

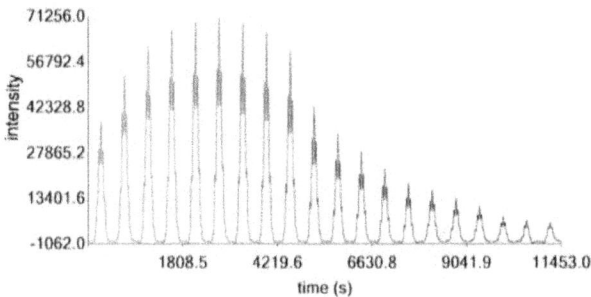

Figure 8. First integral X-band EPR spectrum of virgin olive oil (0.500 g) *vs* time after addition of **1** (100 µL, 7.00 mM) at RT. The time period between two adjacent spectra is 6.5 min.

abovementioned two spectral characteristics as evaluating parameters. The mechanism of the radical initiation by **1** and **2** complexes was further investigated by spin trap experiments.

3.4. Radical traps

The life time of organic free radicals is usually very short because they undergo bimolecular self-reaction. Spin trap technique has been developed since 1968 for the detection and identification of the transient free radicals. Spin traps are diamagnetic molecules exerting a particular high affinity for reactive radicals, to which reactive radicals rapidly add to form persistent spin adducts, detectable in the EPR spectroscopy. Typically, there are two types of molecules serving as spin traps, the C-nitroso compounds and the nitrones; some of them are shown in **Table 1**.

The first one, the C-nitroso compounds are organic nitroxides which upon reaction form the spin adduct through addition of organic part of the radical directly on the nitrogen atom [100, 101]. This proximity to the unpaired electron occupying the p* orbital of N atom of the functional group generates additional hyperfine coupling because of the presence of the neighboring magnetic nuclei of the added free radical. These hyperfine coupling parameters can provide structural information for the identification of added radical. The spin adducts of C-nitroso compounds in general have longer life times but bound less types of radicals, usually the C-centered ones, than nitrones [102]. The second type of spin traps, nitrones are organic molecules reacting with free radicals very fast, close to the diffusion-controlled limit, forming spin adducts by the bound of the added radical to the unsaturated C atom next to the N atom

Table 1. Spin traps commonly used for detection and identification of free radicals.

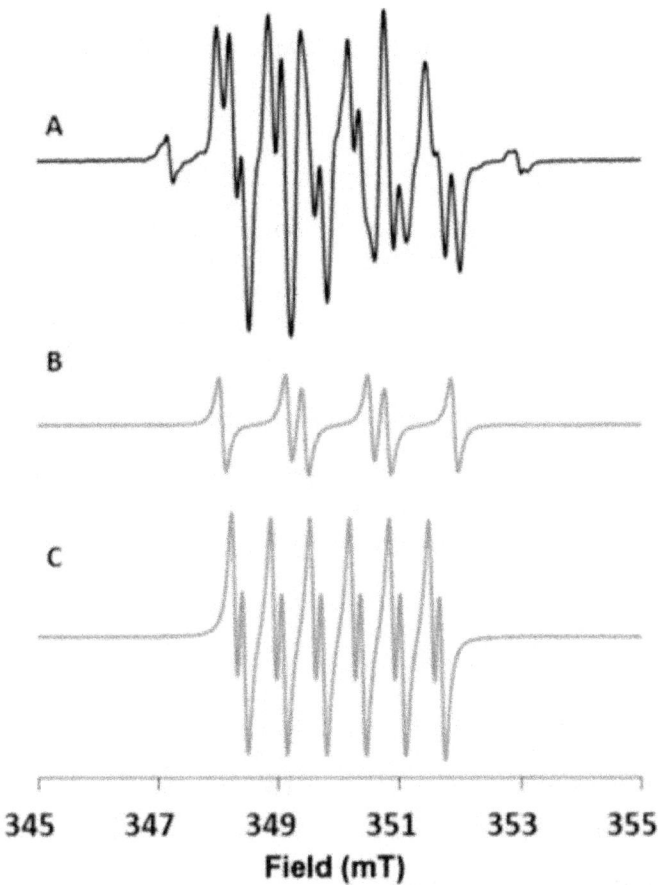

Figure 9. (A) X-band EPR spectra of a solution of 200 μL **1** (7.0 mM, in CH$_2$Cl$_2$) 0.5 g pomace olive oil and 100 μL DMPO (30.0 mM DMPO in CH$_3$OH) at 5 min, (B, C) simulated spectra of the two components of the experimental spectra (A$_N$ = 1.37 and A$_H$ = 1.06 mT (DMPO-OOR) and with A$_N$ = 1.31, A$_{H\beta}$ = 0.65, and A$_{H\gamma}$ = 0.17 mT (DMPO-OR)).

of the functional group [101–103]. It appears that this type of traps is widely used because they can form spin adducts with a wide range of radical species, such as peroxy (HOO$^\bullet$), alkoperoxy (ROO$^\bullet$), alkoxy (RO$^\bullet$), hydroxy (HO$^\bullet$), acyloxy radicals, as well as with other heteroatom-centered radical, including halogen atoms. The prime drawback for this type of traps is the poor information provided by their EPR spectra: the unpaired electron gives hyperfine coupling in the very best cases only from nitrogen nuclei of the function group and the β-proton, but not from the added radical. Thus, identification of the free radical goes through comparison of the under examination EPR spectra with undoubtfully characterized spectra obtained from the spin adducts of the prototype radicals.

An example of the use of DMPO for the detection of the alkoperoxyl and the alkoxyl lipid radicals is shown in **Figure 9**. The spectrum was acquired 5 min after the addition of DMPO, and the vanadium complex **1** in olive oil. Deconvolution of the spectra fits to the alkoperoxyl lipid radical adduct of DMPO (DMPO-OOR) (A$_N$ = 1.37 and A$_H$ = 1.06 mT) in 33%, and the alkoxyl lipid radical adduct of DMPO (DMPO-OR) of (A_N = 1.31, $A_{H\beta}$ = 0.65, and $A_{H\gamma}$ = 0.17 mT) in 77%, and a minor unknown carbon adduct of DMPO (DMPO-CRR'R'').

4. Conclusions

In this chapter, we have reviewed the main cw X-band EPR methodologies used for the study of foods, by observing endogenous unpaired electronic spin species and by the initiation and detection of radicals in foods. The use of EPR for analysis of foods is growing up rapidly. New methodologies in initiation and detection of radicals have resulted in the better understanding of the mechanisms involved in food oxidation processes. The high sensitivity and versatility of EPR makes this technique a valuable tool in food science, and further applications are expected to emerge in the future.

The cw EPR methods used for the characterization of foods are based on the recording of endogenous metal ion or organic radical preexisting in food or the initiation of radicals that can be detected directly or by the addition of radical traps. This chapter is an overview of these methods focusing to the research of the last 15 years.

Acknowledgements

Supported by Research Promotional Foundation of Cyprus and the European Structural Funds ΑΝΑΒΑΘΜΙΣΗ/ΠΑΓΙΟ/0308/32.

Notes/Thanks/Other declarations

The cw X-band EPR spectra in this review were acquired on an ELEXSYS E500 Bruker spectrometer at resonance frequency ~9.5 GHz and modulation frequency 100 MHz. Figures were produced by the software MultiSpecEPR (the software has been developed by Prof. AD Keramidas).

Author details

Chryssoula Drouza[1]*, Smaragda Spanou[1] and Anastasios D. Keramidas[2]

*Address all correspondence to: chryssoula.drouza@cut.ac.cy

1 Department of Agricultural Sciences, Biotechnology and Food Science, Cyprus University of Technology, Limassol, Cyprus

2 Department of Chemistry, University of Cyprus, Nicosia, Cyprus

References

[1] Gómez-Caravaca AM, Maggio RM, Cerretani L. Chemometric applications to assess quality and critical parameters of virgin and extra-virgin olive oil. A review. Analytica Chimica Acta. 2016;**913**:1-21

[2] Siddiqui AJ, Musharraf SG, Choudhary MI, Rahman AU. Application of analytical methods in authentication and adulteration of honey. Food Chemistry. 2017;**217**:687-698

[3] Drouza C, Dieronitou A, Hadjiadamou I, Stylianou M. Investigation of phenols activity in early stage oxidation of edible oils by electron paramagnetic resonance and 19F NMR spectroscopies using novel lipid vanadium complexes as radical initiators. Journal of Agricultural and Food Chemistry. 2017;**65**:4942-4951

[4] Vlasiou M, Drouza C. 19F NMR for the speciation and quantification of the OH-molecules in complex matrices. Analytical Methods. 2015;**7**:3680-3684

[5] Lund A, Shiotani M. Applications of EPR in Radiation Research. Spinger. Switzerland. 2014

[6] Capece A, Romaniello R, Scrano L, Siesto G, Romano P. Yeast starter as a biotechnological tool for reducing copper content in wine. Frontiers in Microbiology. 2018;**8**:**2632**

[7] Drew SC, Robertsa B, Troupb GJ. In Scotch whisky, from where are the Fe^{3+} and Cu^{2+} ions sourced? In: Proceedings—37th Annual Condensed Matter and Materials Meeting; Wagga Wagga, NSW, Australia; 2013

[8] Carreon-Alvarez A, Herrera-Gonzalez A, Casillas N, Prado-Ramirez R, Estarron-Espinosa M, Soto V, de la Cruz W, Barcena-Soto M, Gomez-Salazar S. Cu (II) removal from tequila using an ion-exchange resin. Food Chemistry. 2011;**127**:1503-1509

[9] Rousseva M, Kontoudakis N, Schmidtke LM, Scollary GR, Clark AC. Impact of wine production on the fractionation of copper and iron in Chardonnay wine: Implications for oxygen consumption. Food Chemistry. 2016;**203**:440-447

[10] Morsy MA, Khaled MM. Novel EPR characterization of the antioxidant activity of tea leaves. Spectrochimica Acta Part A: Molecular and Biomolecular Spectroscopy. 2002;**58**: 1271-1277

[11] Hunsicker-Wang L, Vogt M, Derose VJ. EPR methods to study specific metal-ion binding sites in RNA. Methods in Enzymology. 2009;**468**:335-367

[12] Morrissey SR, Horton TE, DeRose VJ. Mn^{2+} sites in the hammerhead ribozyme investigated by EPR and continuous-wave Q-band ENDOR spectroscopies. Journal of the American Chemical Society. 2000;**122**:3473-3481

[13] Goodman BA, Severino JF, Pirker KF. Reactions of green and black teas with Cu(ii). Food & Function. 2012;**3**:399-409

[14] Troup GJ, Navarini L, Liverani FS, Drew SC. Stable radical content and anti-radical activity of roasted Arabica coffee: From in-tact bean to coffee brew. PLoS One. 2015;**10**:e0122834

[15] Stoll S, Schweiger A. EasySpin, a comprehensive software package for spectral simulation and analysis in EPR. Journal of Magnetic Resonance. 2006;**178**:42-55

[16] Klencsár Z, Köntös Z. EPR analysis of Fe^{3+} and Mn^{2+} complexation sites in fulvic acid extracted from lignite. The Journal of Physical Chemistry. A. 2018;**122**:3190-3203

[17] Morsy MA. Teas: Direct test on quality and antioxidant activity using electron paramagnetic resonance spectroscopy. Spectroscopy. 2002;**16**:371-378

[18] Ishigure S, Mitsui T, Ito S, Kondo Y, Kawabe S, Kondo M, Dewa T, Mino H, Itoh S, Nango M. Peroxide decoloration of CI acid orange 7 catalyzed by manganese chlorophyll derivatives at the surfaces of micelles and lipid bilayers. Langmuir. 2010;**26**:7774-7782

[19] Bryliakov KP, Kholdeeva OA, Vanina MP, Talsi EP. Role of MnIV species in Mn(salen) catalyzed enantioselective aerobic epoxidations of alkenes: An EPR study. Journal of Molecular Catalysis A: Chemical. 2002;**178**:47-53

[20] Kaneda H, Kano Y, Koshino S, Ohyanishiguchi H. Behavior and role of iron ions in beer deterioration. Journal of Agricultural and Food Chemistry. 1992;**40**:2102-2107

[21] Jaklová Dytrtová J, Straka M, Bělonožníková K, Jakl M, Ryšlavá H. Does resveratrol retain its antioxidative properties in wine? Redox behaviour of resveratrol in the presence of Cu(II) and tebuconazole. Food Chemistry. 2018;**262**:221-225

[22] Monforte AR, Martins SIFS, Silva Ferreira AC. Strecker aldehyde formation in wine: New insights into the role of gallic acid, glucose, and metals in phenylacetaldehyde formation. Journal of Agricultural and Food Chemistry. 2018;**66**:2459-2466

[23] Pazos M, Da Rocha AP, Roepstorff P, Rogowska-Wrzesinska A. Fish proteins as targets of ferrous-catalyzed oxidation: Identification of protein carbonyls by fluorescent labeling on two-dimensional gels and MALDI-TOF/TOF mass spectrometry. Journal of Agricultural and Food Chemistry. 2011;**59**:7962-7977

[24] Guo A, Kontoudakis N, Scollary GR, Clark AC. Production and isomeric distribution of xanthylium cation pigments and their precursors in wine-like conditions: Impact of Cu (II), Fe(II), Fe(III), Mn(II), Zn(II), and Al(III). Journal of Agricultural and Food Chemistry. 2017;**65**:2414-2425

[25] Clark AC, Wilkes EN, Scollary GR. Chemistry of copper in white wine: A review. Australian Journal of Grape and Wine Research. 2015;**21**:339-350

[26] Danilewicz JC. Chemistry of manganese and interaction with iron and copper in wine. American Journal of Enology and Viticulture. 2016;**67**:377-384

[27] Kreitman GY, Cantu A, Waterhouse AL, Elias RJ. Effect of metal chelators on the oxidative stability of model wine. Journal of Agricultural and Food Chemistry. 2013;**61**:9480-9487

[28] Socha R, Baczkowicz M, Fortuna T, Kura A, Łabanowska M, Kurdziel M. Determination of free radicals and flavan-3-ols content in fermented and unfermented teas and properties of their infusions. European Food Research and Technology. 2013;**237**:167-177

[29] Troup GJ, Hutton DR, Hewitt DG, Hunter CR. Free radicals in red wine, but not in white? Free Radical Research. 1994;**20**:63-68

[30] Goodman BA, Glidewell SM, Arbuckle CM, Bernardin S, Cook TR, Hillman JR. An EPR study of free radical generation during maceration of uncooked vegetables. Journal of the Science of Food and Agriculture. 2002;**82**:1208-1215

[31] Alberti A, Chiaravalle E, Corda U, Fuochi P, Macciantelli D, Mangiacotti M, Marchesani G, Plescia E. Treating meats with ionising radiations. An EPR approach to the reconstruction of the administered dose and its reliability. Applied Radiation and Isotopes. 2011;**69**: 112-117

[32] Alberti A, Chiaravalle E, Fuochi P, Macciantelli D, Mangiacotti M, Marchesani G, Plescia E. Irradiated bivalve mollusks: Use of EPR spectroscopy for identification and dosimetry. Radiation Physics and Chemistry. 2011;**80**:1363-1370

[33] Aleksieva KI, Yordanov ND. Various approaches in EPR identification of gamma-irradiated plant foodstuffs: A review. Food Research International. 2018;**105**:1019-1028

[34] Bercu V, Negut CD, Duliu OG. Irradiation free radicals in freshwater crayfish *Astacus leptodactylus* Esch investigated by EPR spectroscopy. Radiation Physics and Chemistry. 2017;**133**:45-51

[35] Beshir WB. Identification and dose assessment of irradiated cardamom and cloves by EPR spectrometry. Radiation Physics and Chemistry. 2014;**96**:190-194

[36] Bhatti IA, Akram K, Kwon JH. An investigation into gamma-ray treatment of shellfish using electron paramagnetic resonance spectroscopy. Journal of the Science of Food and Agriculture. 2012;**92**:759-763

[37] De Oliveira MRR, Mandarino JMG, Del Mastro NL. Radiation-induced electron paramagnetic resonance signal and soybean isoflavones content. Radiation Physics and Chemistry. 2012;**81**:1516-1519

[38] Della Monaca S, Fattibene P, Boniglia C, Gargiulo R, Bortolin E. Identification of irradiated oysters by EPR measurements on shells. Radiation Measurements. 2011;**46**:816-821

[39] Duliu OG, Bercu V. ESR investigation of the free radicals in irradiated foods. In: Electron Spin Resonance in Food Science. Academic Press. Massachusetts. 2017. pp. 17-32

[40] Yakhin RG, Samigullina NA, Yagund EM, Yakhin RR. Investigation of the influence of microwave radiation on the properties of vegetable food products by methods of EPR and IR spectroscopy. Khimiya Rastitel'nogo Syr'ya. 2017:151-157

[41] Fan D, Liu Y, Hu B, Lin L, Huang L, Wang L, Zhao J, Zhang H, Chen W. Influence of microwave parameters and water activity on radical generation in rice starch. Food Chemistry. 2016;**196**:34-41

[42] Fan DM, Lin LF, Wang LY, Huang LL, Hu B, Gu XH, Zhao JX, Zhang H. The influence of metal ions on the dielectric enhancement and radical generation of rice starch during microwave processing. International Journal of Biological Macromolecules. 2017;**94**:266-270

[43] Lin L, Huang L, Fan D, Hu B, Gao Y, Lian H, Zhao J, Zhang H, Chen W. Effects of the components in rice flour on thermal radical generation under microwave irradiation. International Journal of Biological Macromolecules. 2016;**93**:1226-1230

[44] Walton JC. Functionalised oximes: Emergent precursors for carbon-, nitrogen- and oxygen-centred radicals. Molecules. 2016;**21**:21010063

[45] Hricovíni M, Dvoranová D, Barbieriková Z, Jantová S, Bella M, Šoral M, Brezová V. 6-Nitroquinolones in dimethylsulfoxide: Spectroscopic characterization and photoactivation of molecular oxygen. Journal of Photochemistry and Photobiology A: Chemistry. 2017;**332**: 112-121

[46] Hayes EC, Jian Y, Li L, Stoll S. EPR study of UV-irradiated thymidine microcrystals supports radical intermediates in spore photoproduct formation. The Journal of Physical Chemistry. B. 2016;**120**:10923-10931

[47] Ottaviani MF, Spallaci M, Cangiotti M, Bacchiocca M, Ninfali P. Electron paramagnetic resonance investigations of free radicals in extra virgin olive oils. Journal of Agricultural centred radicals. Molecules. 2016;**21**:21010063

[48] Skoutas D, Haralabopoulos D, Avramiotis S, Sotiroudis TG, Xenakis A. Virgin olive oil: Free radical production studied with spin-trapping electron paramagnetic resonance spectroscopy. Journal of the American Oil Chemists' Society. 2001;**78**:1121-1125

[49] Kurdziel M, Filek M, Łabanowska M. The impact of short-term UV irradiation on grains of sensitive and tolerant cereal genotypes studied by EPR. Journal of the Science of Food and Agriculture. 2018;**98**:2607-2616

[50] Kameya H, Watanabe J, Takano-Ishikawa Y, Todoriki S. Comparison of scavenging capacities of vegetables by ORAC and EPR. Food Chemistry. 2014;**145**:866-873

[51] Kohri S, Fujii H. 2,2′-Azobis(isobutyronitrile)-derived alkylperoxyl radical scavenging activity assay of hydrophilic antioxidants by employing EPR spin trap method. Journal of Clinical Biochemistry and Nutrition. 2013;**53**:134-138

[52] Alvarenga BR, Xavier FAN, Soares FLF, Carneiro RL. Thermal stability assessment of vegetable oils by Raman spectroscopy and chemometrics. Food Analytical Methods. 2018;**11**:1969-1976

[53] Forero-Doria O, García MF, Vergara CE, Guzman L. Thermal analysis and antioxidant activity of oil extracted from pulp of ripe avocados. Journal of Thermal Analysis and Calorimetry. 2017;**130**:959-966

[54] Redondo-Cuevas L, Castellano G, Raikos V. Natural antioxidants from herbs and spices improve the oxidative stability and frying performance of vegetable oils. International Journal of Food Science and Technology. 2017;**52**:2422-2428

[55] Yalcin S, Schreiner M. Stabilities of tocopherols and phenolic compounds in virgin olive oil during thermal oxidation. Journal of Food Science and Technology. 2018;**55**:244-251

[56] Zawadzki A, Alloo C, Grossi AB, do Nascimento ESP, Almeida LC, Bogusz Junior S, Skibsted LH, Cardoso DR. Effect of hop β-acids as dietary supplement for broiler chickens on meat composition and redox stability. Food Research International. 2018;**105**:210-220

[57] Zawada K, Kozłowska M, Zbikowska A. Oxidative stability of the lipid fraction in cookies—The EPR study. Nukleonika. 2015;**60**:469-473

[58] Goodman BA, Pascual EC, Yeretzian C. Real time monitoring of free radical processes during the roasting of coffee beans using electron paramagnetic resonance spectroscopy. Food Chemistry. 2011;**125**:248-254

[59] Yeretzian C, Pascual EC, Goodman BA. Effect of roasting conditions and grinding on free radical contents of coffee beans stored in air. Food Chemistry. 2012;**131**:811-816

[60] Cui L, Lahti PM, Decker EA. Evaluating electron paramagnetic resonance (EPR) to measure lipid oxidation lag phase for shelf-life determination of oils. Journal of the American Oil Chemists' Society. 2017;**94**:89-97

[61] Ricca M, Foderà V, Vetri V, Buscarino G, Montalbano M, Leone M. Oxidation processes in Sicilian olive oils investigated by a combination of optical and EPR spectroscopy. Journal of Food Science. 2012;**77**:C1084-C1089

[62] Cheikhousman R, Zude M, Bouveresse DJR, Léger CL, Rutledge DN, Birlouez-Aragon I. Fluorescence spectroscopy for monitoring deterioration of extra virgin olive oil during heating. Analytical and Bioanalytical Chemistry. 2005;**382**:1438-1443

[63] Silvagni A, Franco L, Bagno A, Rastrelli F. Thermo-induced lipid oxidation of a culinary oil: The effect of materials used in common food processing on the evolution of oxidised species. Food Chemistry. 2012;**133**:754-759

[64] Fundo JF, Miller FA, Tremarin A, Garcia E, Brandão TRS, Silva CLM. Quality assessment of cantaloupe melon juice under ozone processing. Innovative Food Science & Emerging Technologies. 2018;**47**:461-466

[65] Silveira AC, Oyarzún D, Escalona V. Oxidative enzymes and functional quality of mini-mally processed grape berries sanitised with ozonated water. International Journal of Food Science and Technology. 2018;**53**:1371-1380

[66] Zhu F. Effect of ozone treatment on the quality of grain products. Food Chemistry. 2018; **264**:358-366

[67] Łabanowska M, Kurdziel M, Filek M. Changes of paramagnetic species in cereal grains upon short-term ozone action as a marker of oxidative stress tolerance. Journal of Plant Physiology. 2016;**190**:54-66

[68] Reichenauer TG, Goodman BA. Free radicals in wheat flour change during storage in air and are influenced by the presence of ozone during the growing season. Free Radical Research. 2003;**37**:523-528

[69] Mellaerts R, Delvaux J, Levêque P, Wuyts B, G. Van Den Mooter, Augustijns P, Gallez B, Hermans I, Martens J. Screening protocol for identifying inorganic oxides with

anti-oxidant and pro-oxidant activity for biomedical, environmental and food preservation applications. RSC Advances. 2013;**3**:900-909

[70] Moore J, Yin J-J, Yu L. Novel fluorometric assay for hydroxyl radical scavenging capacity (HOSC) estimation. Journal of Agricultural and Food Chemistry. 2006;**54**:617-626

[71] Staško A, Polovka M, Brezová V, Biskupič S, Malík F. Tokay wines as scavengers of free radicals (an EPR study). Food Chemistry. 2006;**96**:185-196

[72] Fadda A, Barberis A, Sanna D. Influence of pH, buffers and role of quinolinic acid, a novel iron chelating agent, in the determination of hydroxyl radical scavenging activity of plant extracts by electron paramagnetic resonance (EPR). Food Chemistry. 2018;**240**: 174-182

[73] Dragišić Maksimović J, Poledica M, Mutavdžić D, Mojović M, Radivojević D, Milivojević J. Variation in nutritional quality and chemical composition of fresh strawberry fruit: Combined effect of cultivar and storage. Plant Foods for Human Nutrition. 2015;**70**:77-84

[74] Pejin B, Savic AG, Petkovic M, Radotic K, Mojovic M. In vitro anti-hydroxyl radical activity of the fructooligosaccharides 1-kestose and nystose using spectroscopic and computational approaches. International Journal of Food Science and Technology. 2014; **49**:1500-1505

[75] Valavanidis A, Nisiotou C, Papageorgiou Y, Kremli I, Satravelas N, Zinieris N, Zygalaki H. Comparison of the radical scavenging potential of polar and lipidic fractions of olive oil and other vegetable oils under normal conditions and after thermal treatment. Journal of Agricultural and Food Chemistry. 2004;**52**:2358-2365

[76] Azman NAM, Peiró S, Fajarí L, Julià L, Almajano MP. Radical scavenging of white tea and its flavonoid constituents by electron paramagnetic resonance (EPR) spectroscopy. Journal of Agricultural and Food Chemistry. 2014;**62**:5743-5748

[77] Atanassova D, Kefalas P, Psillakis E. Measuring the antioxidant activity of olive oil mill wastewater using chemiluminescence. Environment International. 2005;**31**:275-280

[78] Bezzi S, Loupassaki S, Petrakis C, Kefalas P, Calokerinos A. Evaluation of peroxide value of olive oil and antioxidant activity by luminol chemiluminescence. Talanta. 2008;**77**:642-646

[79] Tsiaka T, Christodouleas DC, Calokerinos AC. Development of a chemiluminescent method for the evaluation of total hydroperoxide content of edible oils. Food Research International. 2013;**54**:2069-2074

[80] Kostecka-Gugała A, Ledwozyw-Smoleń I, Augustynowicz J, Wyzgolik G, Kruczek M, Kaszycki P. Antioxidant properties of fruits of raspberry and blackberry grown in Central Europe. Open Chemistry. 2015;**13**:1313-1325

[81] Papadimitriou V, Maridakis GA, Sotiroudis TG, Xenakis A. Antioxidant activity of polar extracts from olive oil and olive mill wastewaters: An EPR and photometric study. European Journal of Lipid Science and Technology. 2005;**107**:512-520

[82] Papadimitriou V, Sotiroudis TG, Xenakis A, Sofikiti N, Stavyiannoudaki V, Chaniotakis NA. Oxidative stability and radical scavenging activity of extra virgin olive oils: An electron paramagnetic resonance spectroscopy study. Analytica Chimica Acta. 2006; **573–574**:453-458

[83] Stavikova L, Polovka M, Hohnová B, Karásek P, Roth M. Antioxidant activity of grape skin aqueous extracts from pressurized hot water extraction combined with electron paramagnetic resonance spectroscopy. Talanta. 2011;**85**:2233-2240

[84] Osorio C, Carriazo JG, Almanza O. Antioxidant activity of corozo (*Bactris guineensis*) fruit by electron paramagnetic resonance (EPR) spectroscopy. European Food Research and Technology. 2011;**233**:103-108

[85] Polak J, Bartoszek M, Chorążewski M. Antioxidant capacity: Experimental determination by EPR spectroscopy and mathematical modeling. Journal of Agricultural and Food Chemistry. 2015;**63**:6319-6324

[86] Polak J, Bartoszek M, Stanimirova I. A study of the antioxidant properties of beers using electron paramagnetic resonance. Food Chemistry. 2013;**141**:3042-3049

[87] Košťálova Z, Hromádková Z, Ebringerová A, Polovka M, Michaelsen TE, Paulsen BS. Polysaccharides from the Styrian oil-pumpkin with antioxidant and complement-fixing activity. Industrial Crops and Products. 2013;**41**:127-133

[88] Bartoszek M, Polak J, Chorążewski M. Comparison of antioxidant capacities of different types of tea using the spectroscopy methods and semi-empirical mathematical model. European Food Research and Technology. 2018;**244**:595-601

[89] Polak J, Bartoszek M. The study of antioxidant capacity of varieties of Nalewka, a traditional Polish fruit liqueur, using EPR, NMR and UV-vis spectroscopy. Journal of Food Composition and Analysis. 2015;**40**:114-119

[90] Aliaga C, López de Arbina A, Rezende MC. "Cut-off" effect of antioxidants and/or probes of variable lipophilicity in microheterogeneous media. Food Chemistry. 2016; **206**:119-123

[91] Balanč BD, Ota A, Djordjević VB, Šentjurc M, Nedović VA, Bugarski BM, Ulrih NP. Resveratrol-loaded liposomes: Interaction of resveratrol with phospholipids. European Journal of Lipid Science and Technology. 2015;**117**:1615-1626

[92] Chatzidaki MD, Arik N, Monteil J, Papadimitriou V, Leal-Calderon F, Xenakis A. Microemulsion versus emulsion as effective carrier of hydroxytyrosol. Colloids and Surfaces B: Biointerfaces. 2016;**137**:146-151

[93] Chatzidaki MD, Mitsou E, Yaghmur A, Xenakis A, Papadimitriou V. Formulation and characterization of food-grade microemulsions as carriers of natural phenolic antioxidants. Colloids and Surfaces A: Physicochemical and Engineering Aspects. 2015;**483**:130-136

[94] Rübe A, Klein S, Mäder K. Monitoring of in vitro fat digestion by electron paramagnetic resonance spectroscopy. Pharmaceutical Research. 2006;**23**:2024-2029

[95] Drouza C, Keramidas AD. Solid state and aqueous solution characterization of rectangular tetranuclear VIV/V-p-semiquinonate/hydroquinonate complexes exhibiting a proton induced electron transfer. Inorganic Chemistry. 2008;**47**:7211-7224

[96] Drouza C, Vlasiou M, Keramidas AD. Vanadium(iv/v)-p-dioxolene temperature induced electron transfer associated with ligation/deligation of solvent molecules. Dalton Transactions. 2013;**42**:11831-11840

[97] Kundu S, Maity S, Weyhermüller T, Ghosh P. Oxidovanadium catechol complexes: Radical versus non-radical states and redox series. Inorganic Chemistry. 2013;**52**:7417-7430

[98] Stylianou M, Drouza C, Giapintzakis J, Athanasopoulos GI, Keramidas AD. Aerial oxidation of a VIV-iminopyridine hydroquinonate complex: A trap for the VIV-semiquinonate radical intermediate. Inorganic Chemistry. 2015;**54**:7218-7229

[99] Adao P, Maurya MR, Kumar U, Avecilla F, Henriques RT, Kusnetsov ML, Pessoa CJ, Correia I. Vanadium-salen and -salan complexes: Characterization and application in oxygen transfer reactions. Pure and Applied Chemistry. 2009;**81**:1279-1296

[100] McCormick ML, Gaut JP, Lin T-S, Britigan BE, Buettner GR, Heinecke JW. Electron paramagnetic resonance detection of free tyrosyl radical generated by myeloperoxidase, lactoperoxidase, and horseradish peroxidase. The Journal of Biological Chemistry. 1998;**273**:32030-32037

[101] Hawkins CL, Davies MJ. Direct detection and identification of radicals generated during the hydroxyl radical-induced degradation of hyaluronic acid and related materials. Free Radical Biology & Medicine. 1996;**21**:275-290

[102] Perkins MJ. Spin trapping. Advances in Physical Organic Chemistry. 1980;**17**:1-64

[103] Venkataraman S, Schafer FQ, Buettner GR. Detection of lipid radicals using EPR. Antioxidants & Redox Signaling. 2004;**6**:631-638

Modeling of Dielectric Resonator Antennas using Numerical Methods Applied to EPR

Sounik Kiran Kumar Dash and Taimoor Khan

Additional information is available at the end of the chapter

http://dx.doi.org/10.5772/intechopen.79087

Abstract

This chapter presents an inclusive analysis of notable techniques carried out on modeling of dielectric resonator (DR)-antenna using numerical methods in last more than two decades. Dielectric resonator antenna (DRA) has created its individual existence in antenna engineering because of its captivating characteristics like; small size, low loss, high efficiency, wide bandwidth, three-dimensional design flexibility as compared to conventional antennas, etc. The DR antennas are being widely modeled using numerical methods nowadays. The triple-folded intention of this chapter is to: (1) give an overview on DRA modeling using single and hybrid numerical methods, (2) give a compressive review of notable numerical modeling researches carried out on DRAs and (3) give some favorable future concentration for the antenna researchers in order to apply the numerical methods on some innovative geometries of DRAs.

Keywords: antennas, dielectric resonator antennas, electromagnetics, microwave, numerical modeling

1. Introduction

The term DR (dielectric resonator)-antenna or some time DRA (dielectric resonator antenna) is derived from dielectric, resonator, and antenna, simultaneously. It is basically an antenna in which a dielectric material resonates at a certain frequency. The word dielectric resonator (DR) was firstly used by Richtmyer [1] long back in mid-1939s. The idea of using DR as a radiating element i.e. antenna in cylindrical shape had been firstly accepted in mid-1983s [2]. DR-antennas have several interesting advantages like; small size, large power handling capacity, less dissipation loss, high efficiency, compatible to any 3-D shape, etc. which make them more popular than that of the traditional antennas. The power handling capability, less loss, and high efficiency are mainly because of the low loss tangent and permittivity of the dielectric resonator while the three-dimensional design flexibility is the function of number of controlling parameters of the resonator's fundamental shapes like; radius for hemispherical shape, height to radius ratio for cylindrical shape and depth/width as well as length/width ratio for rectangular shape [3]. However, because of the advanced simulation and mechanical tools available, different shapes like; hollow cylindrical, conical, hexagonal, triangular, etc. shapes as shown in **Figure 1** are available nowadays.

The mathematical methods used for modeling of DRAs are broadly classified as analytical methods and numerical methods. Up to 1940, the classical methods were widely used for solving the narrow range of electromagnetic (EM) problems only because of complex geometries and mathematical complexities. However, in the mid-1960s, due to the availability of relatively high speed computers, the numerical methods have been supported in their implementation to the EM problems [4]. Since then, numerical methods have taken the place of analytical methods due to numerous advantages, like; lesser computational time, economic for labor purpose, etc. The proposed chapter describes only the three numerical methods: FDTD (finite difference time domain), FEM (finite element method), and MOM (method of moment) which are being widely used for DRAs modeling. In context to this, here different researches carried out on numerical modeling of DRAs in last more than two decades are disused.

2. Dielectric resonator and its antenna characteristics

The gradual development of modern communication systems from microwave-to-millimeter wave had given a chance to Long et al. [2] to investigate dielectric resonator (DR) as a radiator, as a better solution to avoid unnecessary radiation loss, conduction loss, and lower efficiency of conventional microstrip/waveguide antennas at higher frequencies. In course of time, the applications of DRs are not limited to only millimeter but are widely used in microwave and radio frequency ranges also now-a-days. This is because of its several attractive physical characteristics, like 3D-design flexibility, high/low Q-factor, light weight, low cost, ease of excitation, etc. as well as several improved performances in terms of bandwidth, gain, etc. as discussed in the previous section.

Initially, the dielectric resonator was invented in the form of a high Q-factor element specifically used for filters and oscillators [1]. Because of the high Q-factor, the amount of energy stored was much more than the amount of energy lost, which made it to be used as an energy storage device. Once the Q-factor is low, the working is vice versa i.e. the energy radiated is much higher than the energy stored [1]. As per Long et al. [2], when a DR (of low Q-factor) is

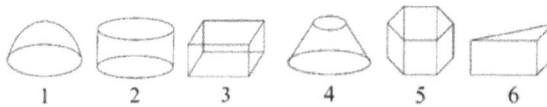

Figure 1. Different geometrical shapes of DR antennas (1—hemispherical, 2—cylindrical, 3—rectangular, 4—conical, 5—hexagonal, and 6—triangular).

placed on a metallic ground surface with unshielded surroundings and an excitation is applied to it, then the discontinuity of the relative permittivity at the resonator surfaces plays an important role. It enables the radio waves bounce back and forth in between the resonator boundary and called as standing electromagnetic wave, means it resonates as well as creates chances of reflection but cannot radiate. It is well known that the resonator walls designed to be transparent to radio waves. Once, the resonator is excited at proper resonating mode, the radio waves start penetrating the resonator boundary and radiate into space. The desired resonating mode can be achieved by proper positioning of dielectric resonator, ground plane, feed, and slot. Moreover, the field distribution inside the resonator as well as the radiation pattern in the space, are distinct depending upon the resonating mode at which the resonator is excited. These modes are mainly divided into three different modes, like transverse electric (TE), transverse magnetic (TM), and hybrid electromagnetic (HEM) modes [3–4]. Generally, for rectangular DRAs, the fundamental modes are considered to be TE_{x111}, TE_{y111}, and TE_{z111}, respectively. For hemispherical DRAs, these are considered as TE_{111} and TM_{101}. Similarly, for cylindrical DRAs, these modes are considered as TE_{01}, TM_{01}, and HE_{11}/EH_{11} [3, 4].

3. FDTD modeling of DRAs

The Finite-Difference-Time-Domain method is one of the popular methods in context of electromagnetic scattering. From historical point of view; the finite difference time domain method was first developed by Yee in 1966 [5]. Later on, it has been extended to electromagnetic three dimensional cases with steady state excitation and also considered to be one of the feasible alternatives to those frequency domain methods. Apart from this, FDTD method has been recognized to be one of the most effective numerical methods in the study of metamaterial-based structures. In 1990, this FDTD method became one of the popular methods of choice for electromagnetic problem analysis, because of several advantages like: ease of understanding, short development time, and explicit type nature [6]. This method has been successfully implemented in different electromagnetic problems like; scattering of antenna (microstrip patch antenna, dielectric resonator antenna), microstrip circuits, etc. However, for the convenience of the readers, few general steps of using FDTD method for DRA modeling are further illustrated in this section.

3.1. Few general steps for FDTD implementation on DRAs

Generally the FDTD method is formulated by considering the differential form of Maxwell's two curl equations which describe the propagation of electric as well as magnetic fields in any medium, which can be uniform, homogeneous, and isotropic. In addition to this, the medium is assumed to be lossless i.e., null volume currents or finite conductivity. Thus, the Maxwell's curl equations can be written as described:

$$\mu \frac{\partial H}{\partial t} = -\nabla \times E \text{ and } \varepsilon \frac{\partial E}{\partial t} = \nabla \times H \tag{1}$$

Here $\mu = \mu_0 \mu_r$ and $\varepsilon = \varepsilon_0 \varepsilon_r$.

For the solution of this type of partial differential equation by FDTD method, a first order finite difference scheme can be used for both time as well as space.

3.2. Step 1: field in time and spatial domain

Let us consider a three dimensional problem as shown in **Figure 2** and define the electric field (or magnetic field) in both space and time domain as [7]:

$$\frac{\partial F(x,y,z,t)}{\partial x} \approx \frac{(F(x+\Delta x/2,y,z,t) - F(x-\Delta x/2,y,z,t))}{\Delta x} = \frac{(F^n(i+0.5,j,k) - F^n(i-0.5,j,k))}{\Delta x}$$

(2)

$$\frac{\partial F(x,y,z,t)}{\partial t} \approx \frac{(F(x,y,z,t+\Delta t/2) - F(x,y,z,t-\Delta t/2))}{\Delta t} = \frac{(F^{n+0.5}(i,j,k) - F^{n-0.5}(i,j,k))}{\Delta t}$$

(3)

As the field is discretized in both space and time domain, hence the practical calculation space is also divided into number of small cubes as shown in **Figure 2(a)**. Here each small cube $\Delta x \times \Delta y \times \Delta z$ of the problem is known as cell size.

3.3. Step 2: Yee's algorithm

For a three-dimensional case, the six field locations are considered as interleaved in space as shown in **Figure 2(b)**. Here each small cells are known as FDTD unit cell [5]. The E-field is calculated at each midpoint of small FDTD cell and for convenience purpose the H-field can be calculated at each spatial locations between two adjacent E-fields.

The field component of x-direction can be written as;

$$H_x^{n+0.5}(i+1,j+0.5,k+0.5) = H_x^{n-0.5}(i+1,j+0.5,k+0.5)$$

$$+\frac{\Delta t}{\mu}\left(\frac{E_y^n(i+1,j+0.5,k+1) - E_y^n(i+1,j+0.5,k)}{\Delta z} - \frac{E_z^n(i+1,j+1,k+0.5) - E_z^n(i+1,j,k+0.5)}{\Delta y}\right)$$

(4)

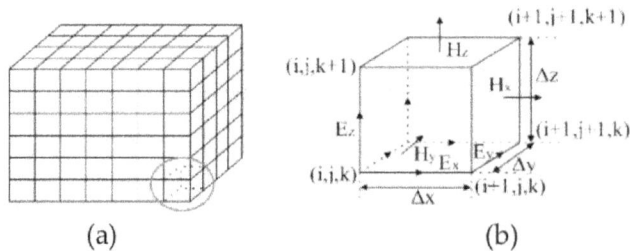

Figure 2. FDTD analysis [7]. (a) FDTD lattice and (b) unit cell.

$$E_x^{n+1}(i+0.5,j,k) = E_x^n(i+0.5,j,k)$$

$$+\frac{\Delta t}{\varepsilon}\left(\frac{H_z^{n+0.5}(i+0.5,j+0.5,k) - H_z^{n+0.5}(i+0.5,j-0.5,k)}{\Delta y} - \frac{H_z^{n+0.5}(i+0.5,j,k+0.5) - H_z^{n+0.5}(i+0.5,j,k+0.5)}{\Delta z}\right)$$

$$(5)$$

Similarly, the field components for y- and z-direction for both electric and magnetic fields can be easily determined. It should be noted here that if the E-field is calculated at nΔt, the H-field is calculated at (n + 0.5)Δt, for which Yee's algorithm is also known as leapfrog algorithm.

3.4. Step 3: estimation of cell size and time step

It is obvious that in FDTD method, finer cell is taken by assuming constant field over a cell. However, the size of the cell depends upon the wavelength of the material. Smaller cell size gives better accuracy. In case of high permittivity dielectric material, the non-homogeneous type cell-size can be used. After fixing the cell-size, the time step can be taken as per Courant-Fricdrich-Lewy stability condition [13].

$$\Delta t \le \frac{1}{v_{max}}\left(\frac{1}{\Delta x^2}+\frac{1}{\Delta y^2}+\frac{1}{\Delta z^2}\right)^{-1/2} \tag{6}$$

Here V_{max} is the maximum phase velocity of the wave in the computational domain/volume. This equation ensures that, error generated in one step does not increase with time marching and using this condition the grid dispersion error can be minimized.

3.5. Step 4: dielectric resonator antenna analysis

A DR-antenna can be a three-dimensional dielectric geometry of any shape along with conducting feed and ground plane. The FDTD method assumes perfect conductor approxima- tion for microstrip line/patch/ground plane whereas perfect dielectric approximation for sub- strate as well as dielectric resonators. In FDTD modeling, the fundamental parameters like; permittivity, permeability, and conductivity are assigned to respective cells in the computa- tional domain to form the objects. Microstrip line/patch/ground plane are generally considered as two-diemensional geometry. Hence the tangential E-field component must be null (0) on the surface. Thus, it can be modeled by applying the boundary conditions on the respective planes of the proper cells. Then, the non-perfect conductor cells like: substrate, dielectric resonator or air, are assigned with respective permittivity (ε_r). For air ε_r will be unity, for substrate and DR the permittivity (ε_r) value can be taken as per the modeling requirement. But for a stacking case, the average value of the interfaces of two/multi dielectric constant can be assigned [7].

3.6. Step 5: source signal and feed modeling

For excitation of the dielectric resonator, the different waveforms like: plane wave, modulated pulse, etc. can be applied. However, in view of smooth waveform, the Gaussian pulse type excitation is preferably used which is mentioned in Eq. (7).

$$p(t) = \begin{cases} e^{-\left[\frac{(t-t_0)}{T_s}\right]^2} & 0 \le t \le 2t_0 \\ 0 & \text{Otherwise} \end{cases} \tag{7}$$

where T_s = spread time, t_0 = peak time.

In practical case, signal is given to the feed line through SMA connector. This feeding in FDTD approach can be modeled by assigning several electric area within the area along the thickness/ height of the substrate which just comes under the strip. Then if the pulse is generated, the fields in the three-dimensional structure can be computed for successive steps until the steady state arrives. Thus, the input impedance (Z_{in}) of the dielectric resonator antenna is calculated easily using Eq. (8)

$$Z_{in}(f) = \frac{V_s(f)}{I_s(f)} \tag{8}$$

where, $V_s(f)$ and $I_s(f)$ are the Fast Fourier Transform (FFT) of the time domain source voltage and source current respectively. Then the return loss can be calculated as:

$$RL_{dB}(f) = 20 \log \left(\frac{Z_{in}(f) - Z_0}{Z_{in}(f) + Z_0} \right) \tag{9}$$

Here Z_0 = 50 Ohm.

3.7. Step 6: boundary conditions

During the analysis of EM problems, it is necessary to truncate the computational domain by a virtual boundary. In addition to this, the boundary should be absorbing one in order to absorb all the radiation to avoid reflection which may causes errors. Hence, it is termed as absorbing boundary condition (ABC) which can be of either Mur's ABC [8] or Berenger's Perfectly Matched Layer (PML) [9]. However, PML is best ABC in terms of accuracy [7].

The above basic steps shows the advancement in computational electromagnetics using FDTD which enabled many researchers for modeling several complex problems based on DRAs. Some notable researches carried out based on this approach in last decade are discussed here.

In 1994, Shum and Luk [10] have analyzed a rectangular DR-antenna fed by a microstrip line through an aperture made on ground plane using FDTD method for calculating the return losses. Again, [11] have analyzed dielectric ring resonator antenna with an air-gap using the FDTD method for improving the impedance bandwidth of the antenna by adjusting the air-gap spacing. A cylindrical dielectric antenna with a dielectric coating has been analyzed using FDTD method for observing the effect of the relative permittivity of the coating material on the impedance bandwidth of the antenna. Then, again [12] have analyzed a cylindrical DRA operating at the fundamental broadside mode using FDTD method for observing the impact of the feed position, probe length, and the dielectric constant on input impedance. Shum and

Luk [13] have presented a FDTD numerical method for modeling probe-fed cylindrical DR antenna for computing the input impedance of the antenna operating in $HEM_{11\delta}$ mode. Chen et al. [14] have analyzed a probe-fed section-spherical DRA using FDTD technique. The mutual coupling between aperture-coupled cylindrical DRAs has been analyzed using FDTD [15]. The aperture-coupled CDRA on a thick ground plane has been investigated using the FDTD method for reducing the coupling from feed-line to the antenna by increasing the thickness of the ground plane [16]. A cross-shaped DRA designed for circular polarization has been analyzed via conformal FDTD method [17]. Kamchouchi and Kayar [18] have demonstrated FDTD method for simplifying the sophisticated radiation problems. Semouchkina et al. [19] have used FDTD method to study the resonant modes in DR-antenna. The in detail study of inter-element coupling phenomena based on a FDTD technique utilizing Berenger's PML boundary conditions and geometrical symmetries has been presented by Gentili et al. [20]. A Microstrip-slot coupled rectangular DRA operated in fundamental TE_{111} mode has been investigated numerically and experimentally [21]. Top-hat monopole antennas loaded with radial layered dielectric has been analyzed using FDTD method for computing input impedance of the antenna structure more accurately [22]. Zhang et al. [23] have investigated a probe-fed DRA element operating in a waveguide environment with application to spatial power combining amplifier arrays using FDTD technique. The radiation pattern and input impedance of the strip-fed rectangular shaped DRA have been computed numerically using FDTD method [24]. Nomura and Sato [25] have proposed a combined method of topology optimization and FDTD method for wideband DR-antenna design. Mohanana et al. [26] have investigated a microstrip line excited compact rectangular DRA using FDTD method. FDTD method has been used to calculate the input impedance of the cylindrical DR-antenna with different dimensions [27]. Li et al. [28] have studied a differentially fed RDRA using FDTD method for the fundamental TE_{111} mode at 2.4 GHz, with a bandwidth of 10.4%. Li and Leung [29] have analyzed a differentially fed rectangular DRA using FDTD method. Thus, the several cases of DRAs have been described using FDTD in this section. Yao et al. [30] have presented an efficient two-dimensional FDTD method for analyzing the parallel-plate dielectric resonator. A Pawn DRA has been investigated in time domain for predicting about 122% impedance bandwidth [31]. Dzulkipli et al. [32] have used a simulation technique based on FDTD to analyze mutual coupling effects in reflectarray environment. Gupta and Gangwar [33] have presented numerical analysis of input impedance, return loss, and radiation characteristics of a strip excited triangular shape DRA (TDRA) using FDTD technique. Thus, several cases based on different shapes of DR-antennas have been successfully resolved.

4. Method of moments for DRAs modeling

Method of moments is sometimes known as moment method (MM). It is considered to be the oldest method in terms of deriving point estimators. The name "method moments" is mainly originated from Russian literature. In western literature, the method of moments has been firstly attributed by Harrington [34], however it became much popular in electromagnetic modeling after the work by Harrington [35]. In course of time MOM has been successfully applied to several practical EM problems like radiation caused by thin-wire elements and arrays, scattering problems, analysis of microstrip and lossy structures and later on for DRA also. So in this context, the modeling of dielectric resonator antenna with some basic steps is clearly discussed in this section. Moreover some published articles of DRA modeling based on this method is also summarized here.

4.1. Few general steps for MOM implementation on DRAs

The integral equations (IE) techniques are quite effective in providing exact solution for dielectric structure modeling. During the modeling of homogeneous system, the integral equations (IE) can be expressed in terms of tangential component of fields (both electric and magnetic) at the media interface only. The equivalence principle [36] is normally used for the solution of scattering problem by using MoM.

4.2. Step 1: representation of field(s) in terms of θ and ϕ

Magnetic field and electric field can be expressed in term of scalar and vector potential by considering position r in θ and ϕ direction for three-dimensional problem as [37]:

$$E_r = \frac{1}{j\omega\varepsilon\mu}\left(\frac{\partial^2}{\partial r^2}+k^2\right)A_r \tag{10}$$

$$E_\theta = \frac{-1}{\varepsilon r\sin\theta}\cdot\frac{\partial F_r}{\partial\phi}+\frac{1}{j\omega\varepsilon\mu r}\cdot\frac{\partial^2 A_r}{\partial r\partial\theta} \tag{11}$$

$$E_\phi = \frac{1}{\varepsilon r}\cdot\frac{\partial F_r}{\partial\theta}+\frac{1}{j\omega\varepsilon\mu r\sin\theta}\cdot\frac{\partial^2 A_r}{\partial r\partial\phi} \tag{12}$$

$$H_r = \frac{1}{j\omega\varepsilon\mu}\left(\frac{\partial^2}{\partial r^2}+k^2\right)F_r \tag{13}$$

$$H_\theta = \frac{1}{\mu r\sin\theta}\cdot\frac{\partial A_r}{\partial\phi}+\frac{1}{j\omega\varepsilon\mu r}\cdot\frac{\partial^2 F_r}{\partial r\partial\theta} \tag{14}$$

$$H_\phi = \frac{-1}{\mu r}\cdot\frac{\partial A_r}{\partial\theta}+\frac{1}{j\omega\varepsilon\mu r\sin\theta}\cdot\frac{\partial^2 F_r}{\partial r\partial\phi} \tag{15}$$

4.3. Step 2: formulation of electric and magnetic potential using Green's function

The electric potential due to a point current J_θ inside and outside the dielectric resonators can be expressed as:

For inside DR (i.e. r < a):

$$G_{J_\theta}^{F_r} = \sum_{n=0}^{\infty} \sum_{m=-n}^{n} A_{nm} P_n^m (\cos \theta) e^{jm\phi} \hat{J}_n (kr) \tag{16}$$

$$G_{J_\theta}^{A_r} = \sum_{n=0}^{\infty} \sum_{m=-n}^{n} B_{nm} P_n^m (\cos \theta) e^{jm\phi} \hat{J}_n (kr) \tag{17}$$

For outside DR (i.e. r > a):

$$G_{J_\theta}^{F_r} = \sum_{n=0}^{\infty} \sum_{m=-n}^{n} C_{nm} P_n^m (\cos \theta) e^{jm\phi} \hat{H}_n (k_0 r) \tag{18}$$

$$G_{J_\theta}^{A_r} = \sum_{n=0}^{\infty} \sum_{m=-n}^{n} D_{nm} P_n^m (\cos \theta) e^{jm\phi} \hat{H}_n (k_0 r) \tag{19}$$

Here the $G_{J_\beta}^{F_r}$ and $G_{J_\beta}^{A_r}$ are the electric potential and magnetic potential in β directed point current, respectively whereas β can be either θ or ϕ. $P_n^m (\cos\theta)$: related to Legendre function of order m and degree n. $\hat{J}_n (kr)$ and $\hat{H}_n (k_0 r)$ represents the spherical Bessel functions of the first kind and spherical Hankel function of the second kind respectively. A_{nm}, B_{nm}, C_{nm}, and D_{nm} can be determined from the boundary condition at the DR-air interface (i.e. r = a) (**Figure 3**).

After applying the boundary condition $E_\theta^+ - E_\theta^- = 0$ as well as $E_\phi^+ - E_\phi^- = 0$ for E-field and $H_\theta^+ - H_\theta^- = 0$ as well as $H_\phi^+ - H_\phi^- = -J_\theta$ ($-J_\theta$ is taken by considering the θ directed current) for H-filed at (r = r' = a) for both θ and ϕ direction four sets of equation relating A_{nm}, B_{nm}, C_{nm}, and D_{nm} can be established, like Eq. (20) (for E-field) and Eq. (21) (for H-field) [37]:

$$\pm K X_{nm} \hat{J}_n (ka) \pm K Y_{nm} \hat{H}_n (k_0 a) = 0 \tag{20}$$

$$\pm K X_{nm} \hat{J}_n (ka) \pm K Y_{nm} \hat{H}_n (k_0 a) = 1 \tag{21}$$

where $\hat{j}_n (ka)$ and $\hat{k}_n (k_0 a)$ are the spherical Bessel function and spherical Henkel function, respectively, K is the ratio of wave number and permittivity, and X_{nm}, Y_{nm} are either A_{nm}, C_{nm} or B_{nm}, D_{nm} [37]. Out of the four sets of equation, by combing the TE mode equations (which

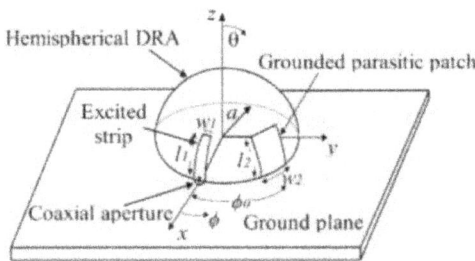

Figure 3. Analysis of hemipsherical DRA [37].

relate to A_{nm}, C_{nm} (in E-field) and B_{nm}, D_{nm} (in H-field)) and TM-mode equation (which relate to B_{nm}, D_{nm} (in E-field) and A_{nm}, C_{nm} (in H-field)) can give a straight forward solution for all four unknowns i.e. A_{nm}, B_{nm}, C_{nm}, and D_{nm}. By putting these values in equation (16-19), the simplified versions of Green's function $G_{J_\theta}^{F_r}$ and $G_{J_\theta}^{A_r}$ can be obtained for both inside (r < a) and outside (r > a) region. Again by applying the similar procedure, the Green's function $G_{J_\phi}^{F_r}$ and $G_{J_\phi}^{A_r}$ for φ directed current can also be obtained.

4.4. Step 3: formulation of E-field and H-field using Green's function

The total E-field because of θ directed and φ directed point currents can be found from potential Green's function. By substituting the values of $G_{J_\theta}^{F_r}$ and $G_{J_\theta}^{A_r}$ (for inside as well as outside cases) in Eqs. (10-15), it can be obtained [37]:

$$G_{J_\theta}^{E_\theta} = \frac{j\eta_0}{2\pi ar} \sum_{n=0}^{\infty} \frac{2n+1}{n(n+1)} \sum_{m=0}^{n} \frac{(n-m)!}{(n+m)!} \cos m(\phi - \phi')$$

$$\times \left\{ \frac{m^2}{\Delta_n^{TE}} \frac{P_n^m(\cos\theta')}{\sin\theta'} \frac{P_n^m(\cos\theta)}{\sin\theta} \Phi_n - \frac{1}{\Delta_n^{TM}\Delta_m} \frac{d}{d\theta} P_n^m(\cos\theta)\psi_n \right\}$$

(22)

Like this $G_{J_\phi}^{E_\phi}$, $G_{J_\phi}^{E_\theta}$ and $G_{J_\phi}^{E_\theta}$ can be obtained [37]. The function Φ_n and ψ_n have different forms for E-field inside (r < a) and outside (r > a) of the dielectric resonator (**Figure 3**). Then with Green's function for the solution of the current (either in the feed probe/feed line/patch/strip etc.) can be found/solved by using MoM.

4.5. Step 4: solution of current using MoM

This Method of Moment solution can be well understood by taking an example (as shown in **Figure 3**). Let in this figure the β (either θ or φ) directed E-field $^AE_{J_\theta}^\beta$, $^BE_{J_\theta}^\beta$, $^BE_{J_\phi}^\beta$ are produced by θ directed excitation strip current J_θ^A, patch current J_θ^B and φ directed patch current J_ϕ^B respectively. Now, by imposing the boundary condition, so that total E-field must vanish on the conducting excitation strip, we get;

$$^AE_{J_\theta}^\theta + {}^BE_{J_\theta}^\theta + {}^BE_{J_\phi}^\theta + E^i = 0$$

(23)

Which can be expressed in terms of Green's functions, i.e.

$$\iint_{S_A} G_{J_\theta}^{E_\theta} J_\theta^A dS' + \iint_{S_B} G_{J_\theta}^{E_\theta} J_\theta^B dS' + \iint_{S_B} G_{J_\phi}^{E_\theta} J_\phi^B dS' + {}^AE^i = 0$$

(24)

Here, S_A and S_B are the surfaces of the excitation strip and parasitic patch respectively, which can further be expressed as:

$$\frac{-1}{W_1}\iint\limits_{S_A} G_{J_\theta}^{E_\theta} I_\theta^A dS' + \frac{-1}{W_2}\iint\limits_{S_B} G_{J_\theta}^{E_\theta} I_\theta^B dS' + \frac{-1}{L_2}\iint\limits_{S_B} G_{J_\phi}^{E_\theta} I_\phi^B dS' = \frac{1}{a}\delta(\theta) \tag{25}$$

Here: $^A E^i = (V_0/a)\delta(\theta)$ and $V_0 = 1$ (unity).

$I_\theta^A = J_\theta^A W_1$, $I_\theta^B = J_\theta^B W_2$, and $I_\phi^B = J_\phi^B L_2$.

Now these currents can be expanded using MoM and resulted as:

$$I_\theta^A(\theta) = \sum_{p_1=1}^{N_1} I_{p_1}^{\theta A} f_{p_1}^{\theta A}(\theta) \tag{26}$$

$$I_\theta^B(\theta) = \sum_{p_2=1}^{N_2} I_{p_2}^{\theta B} f_{p_2}^{\theta B}(\theta) \tag{27}$$

$$I_\phi^B(\theta) = \sum_{p_3=1}^{N_3} I_{p_3}^{\phi B} f_{p_3}^{\phi B}(\phi) \tag{28}$$

where, $f_{p_1}^{\theta A}(\theta)$, $f_{p_2}^{\theta B}(\theta)$, and $f_{p_3}^{\phi B}(\phi)$ are PWS basis functions [38]. Similarly two more equations can be obtained by enforcing the boundary conditions, like;

$$^A E_{J_\theta}^\theta + {}^B E_{J_\theta}^\theta + {}^B E_{J_\phi}^\theta = 0 \tag{29}$$

$$^A E_{J_\theta}^\phi + {}^B E_{J_\theta}^\phi + {}^B E_{J_\phi}^\phi = 0 \tag{30}$$

By applying Galerkin's procedure again we can obtain three sets of equations as of Eqs. (26)–(28). Then the whole equation set can be solved by using the following matrix formulation [4]:

$$\begin{bmatrix} \left[Z_{\theta\theta}^{AA'}(p_1,q_1)\right]_{N_1\times N_1} & \left[Z_{\theta\theta}^{AB'}(p_1,q_2)\right]_{N_1\times N_2} & \left[Z_{\theta\phi}^{AB'}(p_1,q_3)\right]_{N_1\times N_3} \\ \left[Z_{\theta\theta}^{BA'}(p_2,q_1)\right]_{N_2\times N_1} & \left[Z_{\theta\theta}^{BB'}(p_2,q_2)\right]_{N_2\times N_2} & \left[Z_{\theta\phi}^{BB'}(p_2,q_3)\right]_{N_2\times N_3} \\ \left[Z_{\phi\theta}^{BA'}(p_3,q_1)\right]_{N_3\times N_1} & \left[Z_{\phi\theta}^{BB'}(p_3,q_2)\right]_{N_3\times N_2} & \left[Z_{\phi\phi}^{BB'}(p_3,q_3)\right]_{N_3\times N_3} \end{bmatrix} \times \begin{bmatrix} \left[I_{p_1}^{\theta A}\right]_{N_1\times 1} \\ \left[I_{p_2}^{\theta B}\right]_{N_2\times 1} \\ \left[I_{p_3}^{\phi B}\right]_{N_3\times 1} \end{bmatrix} = \begin{bmatrix} \left[V_{q_1}^A\right]_{N_1\times 1} \\ [0]_{N_2\times 1} \\ [0]_{N_3\times 1} \end{bmatrix} \tag{31}$$

After the current vector $\left[I_{p_1}^{\theta A}\right]$ is obtained from Eq. (31), the input impedance can easily be calculated from $Z_{in} = \gamma / \sum_{p_1=1}^{N_1} I_{p_1}^{\theta A} f_{p_1}^{\theta A}(0)$. Further, here $\gamma = 1$ for equivalent spherical DR while 0.5 for hemispherical DR. Then, the remaining current vectors $\left[I_{p_2}^{\theta B}\right]$, $\left[I_{p_3}^{\phi B}\right]$ together along with $\left[I_{p_1}^{\theta A}\right]$ can be used to calculate the radiation fields of dielectric resonator antenna. Thus, few general mathematical steps are discussed here for implementation of method of moments which are quite useful and simple. The use of this method for analyzing some DRAs in last decades is further summarized here.

Analysis of the disk antennas above the grounded dielectric substrate has been carried out using moment method [39]. The input impedance of a cylindrical DRA excited by an aperture slot has been computed using MOM method together with an efficient matrix solution algorithm [40]. Leung and Luk [41] have studied an aperture-coupled hemispherical DRA using MM method for broadside TE_{111} mode. An aperture-coupled hemispherical shaped DR-antenna operating at the end-fire TE_{221} mode has been studied using MOM method together with Green's function [42]. Liu et al. [43] have analyzed a DRA based on the electric and magnetic field integral equations using MM method. The Green function technique together with the MM method has been used to determine the equivalent magnetic current in the slot of slot-fed DRA with/without a backing cavity [44]. Kishk et al. [45] have done a numerical study of split cylindrical DRAs on a conducting ground plane excited by a coaxial probe excited in HEM_{11} and HEM_{12} modes based on MM method. Then MOM-based surface integral equation solver for studying arbitrarily shaped aperture coupled DRAs has been developed [46]. Chow and Leung [47] have investigated the input impedance of the cavity-backed slot-coupled DRA excited by a slender strip using the MM method. The MOM method with piecewise sinusoidal (PWS) basis and testing functions has been used for analyzing a circularly polarized DRA excited by a spiral slot [48]. A rigorous analysis has been done for the excitation of hemispherical type DR-antenna loaded by a circular disk using MOM [49]. Baghaee et al. [50] have analyzed a probe-fed rectangular DRA on a finite ground plane using MOM. A rigorous analysis of the slot-coupled hemispherical dielectric resonator top-loaded by a conducting cap has been presented using MOM [51]. Eshrah et al. [52] have proposed excitation of DRAs by waveguide slots as a substitute to traditionally used excitation mechanism as well as to enhance bandwidth and to control the power coupled to the DRA using MOM method. The coaxial-aperture-fed hemispherical DRA has been analyzed using MOM method [53]. Lam and Leung [54] have analyzed U-slot excited DRA with a baking cavity using the MOM. Ge and Esselle [55] have analyzed the aperture coupled DRA using MOM method. Borowiec et al. [56] have used MOM approach for analyzing a cavity backed, slot excited DRA. Abdulla and Chakraborty [57] have analyzed hemispherical DRA excited with a thick slot at the short circuited end of waveguide using MM method. For a hemispherical DRA, the integral of the admittance matrix corresponding to the homogeneous Green's function has been evaluated by expressing the homogeneous Green's function in terms of a double summation using MM method [58]. Broad wall longitudinal slot coupled hemispherical DRA has been analyzed using MOM [59]. Thus, the moment method has been successfully applied on several cases of DRAs. Thus, several cases of DRAs have been resolved using moment method in this section.

5. Modeling of DRAs using FEM

Engineering domain is one of vastest system, where mathematical model is one of the suitable alternative for describing the behavior of the whole system in a constructive manner. Finite element method is one of those mathematical modeling technique, initially used for structural analysis during 1960–1970s. However its introduction with electromagnetic scattering problems in 1980s is well documented in [60]. Initially it was mainly based on static, quasi-static, and guided wave problems. In course of time this was highly appreciated for microwave and millimeter-wave system optimization as well as for EM radiation means for antenna. In addition to this, the finite element method (FEM) is one of the numerical tool to have the approximate solution which can be used in general purpose computers and thus increased the usability. In FEM, mainly the problems are divided into different sub domains, known as finite element which causes the problem to have many number of finite element patches [61], and in context to this, now this method is considered to be one of the finest method in computational electromagnetics mainly for antenna modeling, with evidence of good number of publications in electromagnetic domain. However the basic steps of modeling of dielectric resonator antenna (three dimensional structure), is discussed in this section.

5.1. Few general steps for FEM implementation on DRAs

The procedure of implementing FEM for modeling of a dielectric resonator antenna is quite different than those for microstrip patch antennas. The way of defining discretization of the finite volume as well as the boundary condition is quite important in FEM modeling. For smooth understanding, the basic approaches of FEM in context of DRA modeling some basic mathematical steps are elaborated here.

5.2. Step 1: formulation of basic fields

For any electromagnetic problem, first we need to define the field. As here DR-antenna is a three dimensional structure, so let us assume a three-dimensional scattering problem as shown in **Figure 4(a)**, having finite volume V with of permittivity ε and permeability μ surrounded by an area of volume V_∞ of permittivity ε_0 and permeability μ_0 at a finite distance of S. When electromagnetic wave input having angular frequency (ω) is applied then it starts scattering. The electromagnetic filed inside the volume V (E_1, H_1) and outside volume V (E_2, H_2) can be written in terms of vector differential wave equations for a source free region [62].

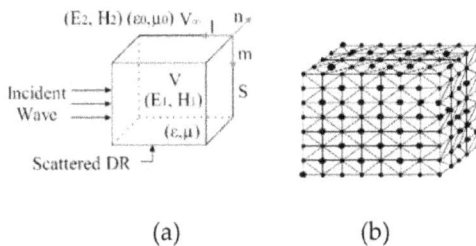

Figure 4. (a) Scattering problem of DRA [62] and (b) discretization of the DR structure [63].

$$\nabla \times \frac{1}{\mu} \nabla \times \overline{E_1} - \omega^2 \varepsilon \overline{E_1} = 0 \tag{32}$$

$$\nabla \times \frac{1}{\varepsilon} \nabla \times \overline{H_1} - \omega^2 \mu \overline{H_1} = 0 \tag{33}$$

$$\nabla \times \nabla \times \overline{E_2} - k_0^2 \overline{E_2} = 0 \tag{34}$$

$$\nabla \times \nabla \times \overline{H_2} - k_0^2 \overline{H_2} = 0 \tag{35}$$

Where K = Free space wave number.

Here three-dimensional FEM can be applied for the solution of fields inside the volume V, whereas a surface integral equation (which is a solution for the fields in V_∞) is then applied to provide a necessary boundary constraint on the surface for the finite element solution. Now, it is the task to solve Eqs. (32) and (33) which is inside the volume, using three-dimensional FEM.

In context of this, the corresponding functional of Eqs. (32) and (33) is highly desired. With little mathematics (using vector identity and applying divergence theorem) the corresponding functional of Eqs. (32) and (33) for the entire domain $V + V_\infty$ can be written as [63]:

$$F = \frac{1}{2}\iiint_V \left[\frac{1}{\omega^2 \mu} (\nabla \times \overline{E_1}) \cdot (\nabla \times \overline{E_1}) - \varepsilon \overline{E_1} \cdot \overline{E_1} \right] dV + \frac{1}{2}\iint_S \frac{1}{\omega^2 \mu} [(\nabla \times \overline{E_1}) \times \overline{E_1}] \cdot \hat{n} dS \tag{36}$$

$$F = \frac{1}{2}\iiint_V \left[\frac{1}{\omega^2 \varepsilon} (\nabla \times \overline{H_1}) \cdot (\nabla \times \overline{H_1}) - \varepsilon \overline{H_1} \cdot \overline{H_1} \right] dV + \frac{1}{2}\iint_S \frac{1}{\omega^2 \varepsilon} [(\nabla \times \overline{H_1}) \times \overline{H_1}] \cdot \hat{n} dS \tag{37}$$

The surface integral in Eqs. (36) and (37) are nearly same and with little mathematics they can be written as:

$$\frac{j}{2\omega}\iint_S [(\overline{E_1} \times \overline{H_1})] \cdot \hat{n} dS \tag{38}$$

Further, in scalar form Eqs. (36) and (37) can be rewritten as:

$$F = \frac{1}{2}\iiint_V \left\{ \frac{1}{\omega^2 \mu} \left[\left(\frac{\partial E_z}{\partial y} - \frac{\partial E_y}{\partial z}\right)^2 + \left(\frac{\partial E_x}{\partial z} - \frac{\partial E_z}{\partial x}\right)^2 + \left(\frac{\partial E_y}{\partial x} - \frac{\partial E_x}{\partial y}\right)^2 \right] - \varepsilon \left[E_x^2 + E_y^2 + E_z^2 \right] \right\} dV$$

$$+ \frac{j}{2\omega}\iint_S (E_l H_m - E_m H_l) dS$$

$$\tag{39}$$

$$F = \frac{1}{2}\iiint_V \left\{ \frac{1}{\omega^2 \varepsilon} \left[\left(\frac{\partial H_z}{\partial y} - \frac{\partial H_y}{\partial z}\right)^2 + \left(\frac{\partial H_x}{\partial z} - \frac{\partial H_z}{\partial x}\right)^2 + \left(\frac{\partial H_y}{\partial x} - \frac{\partial H_x}{\partial y}\right)^2 \right] - \mu \left[H_x^2 + H_y^2 + H_z^2 \right] \right\} dV$$

$$+ \frac{j}{2\omega}\iint_S (E_l H_m - E_m H_l) dS$$

$$\tag{40}$$

Here, the subscript 1 on both E and H has been dropped for convince. Also, l and m are two orthogonal unit vectors tangential to the surface S and they are so oriented that (l, m, n) form a right handed systems.

5.3. Step 2: finite element discretization and surface integral formulation for fields

The finite volume V of the DR can be subdivided into numbers of three-dimensional elements which can be either tetrahedral, rectangular prisms, or a triangular prisms or even better isotropic elements [63] (as shown in **Figure 4(b)**) that depends upon the applications and geometry type. However, within each element the field can be expressed as;

$$\overline{E}^e = \sum_{i=1}^{n} N_i^e(x,y,z)\overline{E}_i^e \text{ and } \overline{H}^e = \sum_{i=1}^{n} N_i^e(x,y,z)\overline{H}_i^e \tag{41}$$

Here; n is the number of nodes, N_i^e is the interpolation function, and $\overline{E}_i^e, \overline{H}_i^e$ in the fields at the ith node.

Substituting Eq. (41) into Eq. (39) or Eq. (40) and applying Rayleigh-Ritz procedure the system of liner equations can be obtained [62]. Now applying three-dimensional finite element discretization to Eq. (39) results in the matrix equation;

$$\left[\overline{\overline{K}}_{II}\right] \cdot \{\overline{E}_I\} + \left[\overline{\overline{K}}_{IS}\right] \cdot \{\overline{E}_S\} = 0 \tag{42}$$

and

$$\left[\overline{\overline{K}}_{II}\right] \cdot \{\overline{E}_{II}\} + \left[\overline{\overline{K}}_{SS}\right] \cdot \{\overline{E}_S\} + \left[\overline{\overline{K}}_{SS}'\right] \cdot \{\overline{H}_S\} = 0 \tag{43}$$

where $\overline{E}_I$ is the electric field nodes interior to the surface S; $\overline{E}_S$ is the tangential electric field at the nodes on S; $\overline{H}_S$ is the tangential magnetic field at the nodes on S, $\overline{\overline{K}}$ is the matrix having three dimensions.

In close observation to Eqs. (41) and (42), it is clear that, they do not form a complete system and this can be achieved by developing matrix equation relating to $\{\overline{E}_S\}$ and $\{\overline{H}_S\}$, hence the Finite element surface integral formulation can be applied as follows:

For a finite domain V bounded by a surface S, the electric field and magnetic field inside, in the form of incident electric field can be expressed as [62]:

$$\overline{E}(\overline{R}) = \overline{E}^{INC}(\overline{R}) - \iint_S \left\{\nabla \times \overline{\overline{G}}_0\left(\overline{R},\overline{R}'\right) \cdot \left[\hat{n}' \times \overline{E}\left(\overline{R}'\right)\right] - j\omega\mu\overline{\overline{G}}_0\left(\overline{R},\overline{R}'\right) \cdot \left[\hat{n}' \times \overline{H}\left(\overline{R}'\right)\right]\right\}dS' \tag{44}$$

After discretizing the above equation on the surface S, a matrix equation comes in the form:

$$\left[\overline{\overline{B}}_{SS}\right] \cdot \{\overline{E}_S\} + \left[\overline{\overline{B}}_{SS}'\right] \cdot \{\overline{H}_S\} = \{\overline{E}_S^{INC}\} \tag{45}$$

where $\overline{E}_S^{INC}$ is the tangential incident electric field at the node on S, and again $\overline{\overline{B}}$ denotes a matrix of three dimensions. Now the combination of Eqs. (42), (43), and (45) form a complete system in order to solve the nodal fields.

For modeling of DRAs, these basic steps of FEM method has also been utilized but the referenced literature on it is very much limited. However some of the collected articles are discussed here. Fargeot et al. [64] have used DR antenna with a non-destructive method based on FEM for characterizing material. A microstrip-coupled cylindrical DRA excited in the $HE_{11\delta}$ mode has been investigated theoretically as well as experimentally using FEM [65]. Neshati and Wu [66] have proposed a microstrip-slot coupled rectangular DRA using FEM. A probe fed rectangular DRA supported by finite ground plane and operated in TE_{111} mode has been analyzed numerically using FEM method [67]. Analysis of waveguide fed DRA has been carried out using FEM [68].

6. Hybrid numerical methods for DRAs modeling

The basic steps for FDTD, MoM, and FEM have well discussed in previous sections. However, in this section several cases of DRAs modeling have been discussed using a combination of more than one numerical method like: combination of MOM with others methods and the combination of FEM with others methods, respectively.

The moment method (MM) has been combined with FDTD for analyzing a rectangular DRA over a finite ground plane with microstrip slot excitation [69] and for analyzing a DRA fed by a microstrip line coupled with DR through a narrow aperture in a ground plane [70], respectively. Again, the moment method has been combined with mode matching method for studying the scattering problem of the probe-fed hemispherical DR antenna utilizing a conducting conformal strip excitation operated in the fundamental TE_{111} mode [71]. A new excitation scheme employing a conducting conformal strip has been analyzed for DRA excitation operated in fundamental mode TE_{111} using mode-matching method [72].

Few cases of DRAs have also been modeled using a combination of FEM and other numerical methods, which are discussed here. The hybrid combination of FEM and conventional dielectric waveguide model (CDWM) has been used for studying a probe-fed rectangular DRA supported by a ground plane theoretically and experimentally, simultaneously [73]. The FEM has again been combined with finite integral method (FIT) for analyzing a novel "C"-shaped DRA [74] as well for reducing the mutual coupling between two identical cylindrical DRAs [75] mounted on a conducting hollow circular cylindrical structure in E-plane and H-plane coupling, respectively. A reflectarray mounted on or embedded in cylindrical and spherical surfaces has been analyzed using finite integration method and transmission line method at 11.5 GHz for satellite applications [76]. Again Dhouib et al. [77] have reported the analysis of aperture-coupled and microstrip proximity coupled DRAs using transmission line method. A hybrid combination of FEM and finite integration method (FIT) has also been used for analyzing an electrically small and high permittivity "C" DRA [78]. The FEM has been combined with FDTD for designing multi-segment DRA [79] and for structural mechanics analysis of DRAs [80], respectively.

7. Electron paramagnetic resonance resonator types and effects

In general electron paramagnetic resonance (EPR) is a spectroscopy tool used in different emerging areas of physics, chemistry, and biology for the characterization of paramagnetic species [81–83]. In general there are some specific types of EPR resonators, say wave-guide resonator, microstrip resonator, dielectric resonator, and transmission line resonator [83]. Unlike traditional EPR wave-guide cavities operating in the transverse electric TE mode, on which both longitudinal and transverse dimensions scale with frequency, transmission-line resonators operating in the transverse electromagnetic (TEM) mode have their resonant frequency set only by the longitudinal dimension and the effective relative permittivity of the medium (εref) which ultimately results in shorter transverse dimensions than half wavelength [84]. As per [85] the conventional EPR systems i.e. using wave guide cavities as well inductive detection have a sensitivity limitation to near 10^{11} spins/GHz$^{1/2}$, which is inadequate for studying samples having smaller number of spins. On the other hand if we see, dielectric resonators (DR) which are made of a single crystal/ceramic material with comparatively high dielectric constants with low loss have better sensitivity of EPR than those conventional ones. It can also achieve sensitivity nearly 5×10^8 spins/G [85]. Apart from this, the small size of the DR also helps in using it as the central part of mini-EPR, while the absence of background signals gives more degrees of freedom for precise recordings of EPR spectra. As per [85] different kind of shapes can be actualized in a DR in order to store and analyze samples. It can be noted that more no of shapes helps in storing and analyzing more number of samples simultaneously. However the modeling work of making different types of shapes as well as their effect on resonator characteristics can be well developed by the numerical methods discussed in previous sections.

Author details

Sounik Kiran Kumar Dash[1] and Taimoor Khan[2]*

*Address all correspondence to: ktaimoor@gmail.com

1 CHRIST (Deemed to be University), Bengaluru, Karnataka, India

2 National Institute of Technology Silchar, Silchar, Assam, India

References

[1] Richtmyer RD. Dielectric resonators. Journal of Applied Physics. Jun. 1939;**10**:391-398

[2] Long SA, Mcallister MW, Shen LC. The resonant cylindrical dielectric cavity antenna. IEEE Transactions on Antennas and Propagation. May 1983;**31**(3):406-412

[3] Mongia RK, Bhartia P. Dielectric resonator antennas—A review and general design relations for resonant frequency and bandwidth. International Journal of Microwave and Millimeter-Wave Computer-Aided Engineering. Jul. 1994;**4**(3):230-247

[4] Dash SKK, Khan T, De A. Modelling of dielectric resonator antennas using numerical methods: A review. Journal of Microwave Power and Electromagnetic Energy. 2016;**50**(4): 269-293

[5] Yee KS. Numerical solution of boundary value problems involving Maxwell's equation in isotropic media. IEEE Transactions on Antennas and Propagation. 1966;**14**:302-307

[6] Inan US, Marshall RA. Numerical Electromagnetics: The FDTD Method. Cambridge: Cambridge University Press; 2011

[7] Kumar AVP. Development of a novel wideband cylindrical dielectric resonator antenna [PhD dissertation]. Cochin, India: Dept. of Electronics, Cochin Univ. of Science and Tech; 2008 Jan

[8] Mur G. Absorbing boundary condition for the finite-difference approximation of the time-domain electromagnetic field equations. IEEE Transactions on Electromagnetic Compatibility. 1981;**23**:377-382

[9] Berenger JP. A perfectly matched layer for the absorption of electromagnetic waves. Journal of Computational Physics. 1994;**114**:185-200

[10] Shum SM, Luk KM. Characteristics of dielectric ring resonator antenna with an air gap. IET Electronics Letters. Feb. 1994;**30**(4):277-278

[11] Shum SM, Luk KM. Numerical study of a cylindrical dielectric-resonator antenna coated with a dielectric layer. IEEE Transactions on Antennas and Propagation. Apr. 1995;**142**(2): 189-191

[12] Shum SM, Luk KM. FDTD analysis of probe-fed cylindrical dielectric resonator operating in fundamental broadside mode. IET Electronics Letters. Jul. 1995;**31**(15):1210-1212

[13] Shum SM, Luk KM. FDTD analysis of probe-fed cylindrical dielectric resonator antenna. IEEE Transactions on Antennas and Propagation. Mar. 1998;**46**(3):325-333

[14] Twu Chen H, Cheng YT, Ke SY. Probe-fed section-spherical dielectric resonator antennas. In: Proceedings of the IEEE Asia Pacific Microwave Conference, vol. 2. Nov. 1999. pp. 359-362

[15] Guo YX, Luk KM, Leung KW. Mutual coupling between rectangular dielectric resonator antennas by FDTD. IEE Proceedings—Microwaves, Antennas and Propagation. Aug. 1999;**146**(4):292-294

[16] Guo YX, Luk KM, Leung KW. Characteristics of aperture-coupled cylindrical dielectric resonator antennas on a thick ground plane. IEE Proceedings—Microwaves, Antennas and Propagation. Dec. 1999;**146**(6):439-442

[17] Farahat N, Yul W, Mittra R, Koleck T. Cross-shaped dielectric resonator antenna analysis using the conformal finite difference time domain (CFDTD) method. In: Proc. IEEE Antennas and Propagation Society Int. Sym, vol. 3; Boston, MA, USA. Jul. 2001. pp. 549-552

[18] Kamchouchi HE, EI-Kayar YG. Finite difference time domain solutions for the dielectric resonator antenna problems with different feeding signals. In: Proc. IEEE 18th Nat. Radio Science Conf; Mansoura. Mar. 2001. pp. 63-70

[19] Semouchkina E, Semouchkin G, Caol W, Mittra R. FDTD analysis of modal characteristics of dielectric resonator antennas. In: Proc. IEEE Antennas and Propagation Society Int. Sym. Vol. 4. 2002. pp. 466-469

[20] Gentili GB, Morini M, Selleri S. Relevance of coupling effects on DRA array design. IEEE Transactions on Antennas and Propagation. Mar. 2003;**51**(3):399-405

[21] Neshati MH, Wu Z. Microstrip-slot coupled rectangular dielectric resonator antenna: Theoretical modelling & experiments. In: Proc. IET 12th Int. Conf. on Antennas and Propagation; March 2003, Conf. Pub. No. 491. Vol. 2. pp. 759-762

[22] Paran K, Kamyab M, Tabatabaei NA. FDTD analysis of top-hat monopole antennas loaded with radially layered dielectric. International Journal of Engineering-Transactions A: Basics. 2004;**17**(3):251-262

[23] Zhang Y, Kishk AA, Yakovlev AB, Glisson AW. FDTD analysis of a probe-fed dielectric resonator antenna in rectangular waveguide. In: Proc. IEEE/ACES Int. Conf. on Wireless Communications and Applied Computational Electromagnetics. Apr. 2005. pp. 371-375

[24] EI-Deen E, Zainud-Deen SH, Sharshar HA, Binyamin MA. The effect of the ground plane shape on the characteristics of rectangular dielectric resonator antennas. In: Proc. IEEE Antennas and Propagation Society Int. Sym; Albuquerque, NM. Jul. 2006. pp. 3013-3016

[25] Nomura T, Sato K. Topology design optimization of dielectric resonator antennas using finite-difference time-domain method. In: Proc. IEEE Antennas and Propagation Society Int. Sym; Albuquerque, NM. Jul. 2006. pp. 1317-1320

[26] Mohanana P, Mridula S, Paul B, Suma MN, Bijumon PV, Sebastian MT. FDTD analysis of rectangular dielectric resonator antenna. Journal of the European Ceramic Society. 2007;**27** (8–9):2753-2757

[27] Zainud-Deen SH, EI-Doda SI, Awadalla KH, Sharshar HA. The relation between lumped-element circuit models for cylindrical dielectric resonator and antenna parameters using MBPE. Progress in Electromagnetics Research. 2008;**1**:79-93

[28] Li A, Leung KW, Sheng XQ. Differentially fed rectangular dielectric resonator antenna. In: Proc. IEEE Global Symp. on Millimeter Waves; Nanjing. Apr. 2008. pp. 157-160

[29] Li B, Leung KW. On the differentially fed rectangular dielectric resonator antenna. IEEE Transactions on Antennas and Propagation. Feb. 2008;**56**(2):353-359

[30] Yao B, Zheng Q, Peng J, Zhong R, Li S, Xiang T. An efficient 2-D FDTD method for analysis of parallel-plate dielectric resonators. IEEE Antennas and Wireless Propagation Letters. Aug. 2011;**10**:866-868

[31] Ganguly D, Das S, Rojatkar A, Guha D. Ultra-wideband pawn DRA: Time domain studies. In: Proc. IEEE Indian Antenna Week; Kolkata. Dec. 2011. pp. 1-4

[32] Dzulkipli NI, Jamaluddin MH, Gillard R, Sauleau R, Ngah R, Kamarudin MR, et al. Mutual coupling analysis using FDTD for di- electric resonator antenna reflectarray radiation prediction. Progress in Electromagnetics Research B. 2012;**41**:121-136

[33] Gupta A, Gangwar RK. Analysis of conformal strip feed triangular dielectric resonator antenna using FDTD method. In: Proc. IEEE Int. Conf. on Computational Electromagnetics; Hong Kong. Feb. 2015. pp. 92-94

[34] Harrington RF. Field Computation by Moment Methods. Malabar, FL: Krieger; 1968

[35] Harrington RF. Matrix methods for field problems. Proceedings of the IEEE. 1967;**55**: 136-149

[36] Harrington RF. Time Harmonic Electromagnetic Fields. New York: McGraw-Hill; 1961

[37] Ng HK. Rigorous analysis of the hemispherical dielectric resonator antenna with a parasitic patch [PhD dissertation]. Hong Kong: Dept. of Electronics Engg. City Univ; Oct 2003

[38] Leung KW, Ng HK. Dielectric resonator antenna fed by displaced conformal strip. Microwave and Optical Technology Letters. 2001;**29**:185-187

[39] Kishk AA, Zunoubi MR. Analysis of the dielectric disc antennas above a grounded dielectric substrate. In: Proc. IEEE Antennas and Propagation Society Int. Symp. Dig; Chicago, IL, USA. Jun 1992. pp. 2171-2174

[40] Junker JP, Kishk AA, Glisson AW. Input impedance of an aperture coupled dielectric resonator antenna. In: Proc. IEEE Antennas and Propagation Society Int. Symp. Dig; Seattle, WA, USA. Jun 1994. pp. 748-751

[41] Leung KW, Luk KM. Moment method solution of aperture-coupled hemispherical dielectric resonator antenna. In: Proc. IEEE Antennas and Propagation Society Int. Symp. Dig., vol. 2; Seattle, WA, USA. Jun. 1994. pp. 752-755

[42] Leung KW, Luk KM. Moment method solution of aperture-coupled hemispherical dielectric resonator antenna using exact modal Green's function. IEE Proceedings - Microwaves, Antennas and Propagation. Oct. 1994;**141**(5):377-381

[43] Liu Z, Hewa WH, Michielssen NDE. Moment method based analysis of dielectric-resonator antennas. In: Proc. IEEE Antennas and Propagation Society Int. Symp., vol. 2; Orlando, FL, USA. Jul. 1999. pp. 806-809

[44] Chow KY, Leung KW, Luk KM, Yung EKN. Input impedance of the slot-fed dielectric resonator antenna with/without a backing cavity. IEEE Transactions on Antennas and Propagation. Feb. 2001;**49**(2):307-309

[45] Kishk A, Glisson AW, Junker GP. Bandwidth enhancement for split cylindrical dielectric resonator antenna. Progress in Electromagnetics Research. 2001;**33**:97-118

[46] Liu Z, Chew WC, Michielssen E. Numerical modeling of dielectric-resonator antennas in a complex environment using the method of moments. IEEE Transactions on Antennas and Propagation. Jan. 2002;**50**(1):79-82

[47] Chow KY, Leung KW. Cavity-backed slot-coupled dielectric resonator antenna excited by a narrow strip. IEEE Transactions on Antennas and Propagation. 2002;**50**:404-405

[48] Qian ZH, Leung KW, Chen RS. Analysis of circularly polarized dielectric resonator antenna excited by a spiral slot. Progress in Electromagnetics Research. 2004;**47**:111-121

[49] Ng HK, Leung KW. Frequency tuning of the dielectric resonator antenna using a loading disk. In: Proc. IEEE Antennas and Propagation Society Int. Symp, vol. 1. Jun. 2004. pp. 1086-1089

[50] Baghaee RM, Neshati MH, Mohassel JR. Moment method analysis of probe-fed rectangular dielectric resonator antennas with a rigorous source modeling and finite ground plane. In: Proc. IEEE Asia-Pacific Conf., vol. 5. Dec. 2005. pp. 4-7

[51] Ng HK, Leung KW. Frequency tuning of the dielectric resonator antenna using a loading cap. IEEE Transactions on Antennas and Propagation. Mar. 2005;**53**(3):1229-1232

[52] Eshrah IA, Kishk AA, Yakovlev AB, Glisson AW. Theory and implementation of dielectric resonator antenna excited by a waveguide slot. IEEE Transactions on Antennas and Propagation. Jan. 2005;**53**(1):483-494

[53] Leung KW, So KK. Analysis of the coaxial-aperture-fed dielectric resonator antenna. In: Proc. IEEE Antennas and Propagation Society Int. Symp.; Albuquerque, NM. Jul. 2006. pp. 2503-2506

[54] Lam HY, Leung KW. Analysis of U-slot-excited dielectric resonator antennas with a backing cavity. IEE Proceedings - Microwaves, Antennas and Propagation. Oct. 2006; **153**(5):480-482

[55] Ge Y, Esselle KP. The analysis of a rectangular dielectric resonator antenna using the method of moments. In: Proc. IEEE Antennas and Propagation Society Int. Symp.; Salt Lake City, UT, USA. Vol. 3. Jul. 2000. pp. 1454-1457

[56] Borowiec R, Kucharski AA, Slobodzian PM. Slot excited dielectric resonator antenna above a cavity - Analysis and experiment. In: Proc. IEEE Int. Conf. on Microwaves, Radar & Wireless Communications; Krakow. May 2006. pp. 824-827

[57] Abdulla P, Chakraborty A. Rectangular waveguide-fed hemispherical dielectric resonator antenna. Progress in Electromagnetics Research. 2008;**83**:225-244

[58] Kakade AB, Ghosh B. Efficient technique for the analysis of microstrip slot coupled hemispherical dielectric resonator antenna. IEEE Antennas and Wireless Propagation Letters. 2008;**7**:332-336

[59] Abdulla P, Singh YK, Chakraborty A. Theoretical and experimental study on broad wall slot coupled dielectric resonator antennas. In: Proc. IEEE Asia Pacific Microwave Conf.; Singapore. Dec. 2009. pp. 2750-2753

[60] Jin JM. The Finite Element Method in Electromagnetics. New York: John Wiley & Sons Inc; 1993

[61] Kwon YW, Bang HC. The Finite Element Method Using MATLAB. New York: CRC Press; 1997. ISBN 0-8493-9653-0

[62] Jin J, Liepa VV, Volakis JL. Finite Element Methods for Electromagnetic Scattering. Ann Arbor, MI: Radiation Lab., Dept. of Elect Eng and Comp Science, The Univ. of Michigan; 1989 Oct. p. 868

[63] Zienkiewicz OC, Taylor RL, Zhu JZ. The Finite Element Method: Its Basis and Fundamentals. Burlington, MA: Elsevier Butterworth-Heinemann; 2005

[64] Fargeot S, Julien-Vergonjanne A, Guillon P. Dielectric resonator antenna for material characterization. In: Proc. IEEE Conf. on Precision Electromagnetic Measurements Dig; Braunschweig, Germany. Jun. 1996. pp. 70-71

[65] Drossos G, Wu Z, Davis LE. Theoretical and experimental investigations on a microstrip-coupled cylindrical dielectric resonator antenna. Microwave and Optical Technology Letters. Apr. 1999;**21**(1):18-25

[66] Neshati MH, Wu Z. Finite element analysis & experimental studies of microstrip slot coupled rectangular dielectric resonator antenna. In: Proc. IEEE Int. Conf. on Microwave and Millimeter Wave Technology. Aug. 2004. pp. 118-121

[67] Neshati MH, Wu Z. Numerical modeling and experimental study of probe-fed rectangular dielectric resonator antenna (RDRA) supported by finite circular ground plane. International Journal of Engineering-Transactions A: Basics. Sept. 2004;**17**(3):269-280

[68] Sheng XQ, Leung KW, Yung EKN. Analysis of waveguide-fed dielectric resonator antenna using a hybrid finite element method/moment method. IEE Proceedings - Microwaves, Antennas and Propagation. Feb. 2004;**151**(1):91-95

[69] Shin J, Kishk AA, Glisson AW. Analysis of rectangular dielectric resonator antennas excited through a slot over a finite ground plane. In: Proc. IEEE Antennas and Propagation Society Int. Symp; Salt Lake City, UT, USA. Vol. 4. Jul. 2000. pp. 2076-2079

[70] Ge Y, Esselle KP. Microwave dielectric-resonator antenna analysis and design. In: Proc. IEEE Asia Pacific Microwave Conf; Sydney, NSW. Dec. 2000. pp. 1473-1476

[71] Chen ZN, Leung KW, Luk KM, Yung EKN. Electromagnetic scattering from the probe-fed hemispherical dielectric resonator antenna. In: Proc. IEEE Antennas and Propagation Society Int. Symp. Dig., vol. 2; Baltimore, MD, USA. Jul. 1996. pp. 1410-1413

[72] Leung KW. Conformal strip excitation of dielectric resonator antenna. IEEE Transactions on Antennas and Propagation. Jun. 2000;**48**(6):961-967

[73] Neshati MH, Wu Z. Rectangular dielectric resonator antennas: Theoretical modelling and experiments. In: Proc. IEE Int. Conf. on Antennas and Propagation, vol. 2; Manchester. Apr. 2001. pp. 866-870

[74] Rotaru MD, Sykulski JK. Design and analysis of a novel compact high permittivity dielectric resonator antenna. IEEE Transactions on Magnetics. Mar. 2009;**45**(3):1052-1055

[75] Zainud-Deen SH, Malhat HA, Awadalla KH. Reduction of mutual coupling between two dielectric resonator antennas mounted on a circular cylindrical ground plane. In: Proc. IEEE Antennas and Propagation Society Int. Symp.; Toronto, ON. Jul. 2010. pp. 1-4

[76] Zainud-Deen SH, EI-Shalaby NA, Malhat HA, Gaber SM, Awadalla KH. Dielectric resonator antenna reflector—Rays mounted on or embedded in conformal surfaces. Progress in Electromagnetics Research C. 2013;**38**:115-128

[77] Dhouib A, Stubbs MG, Mongia RK, Lecours M. TLM analysis of rectangular dielectric resonator antennas. In: Proc. IEEE Antennas and Propagation Society Int. Symp. Dig., vol 1; Newport Beach, CA, USA. Jun. 1995. pp. 782-785

[78] Rotaru M, Sykulski JK. Numerical investigation on compact multimode dielectric resonator antennas of very high permittivity. IET Science, Measurement and Technology. May 2009;**3**(3):217-228

[79] Rashidian A, Forooraghi K, Tayefeh MR. Design algorithm of multi-segment dielectric resonator antennas (MSDRAs). In: Proc. IEEE Int. Conf. on Microwave and Millimeter Wave Technology. Aug. 2004. pp. 134-137

[80] Nomura T, Sato K, Nishiwaki S, Yoshimura M. Topology optimization of multiband dielectric resonator antennas using finite-difference time-domain method. In: Proc. IEEE International Workshop on Antenna Technology: Small and Smart Antennas Metamaterials and Applications; Cambridge. Mar. 2007. pp. 147-150

[81] Geifman IN, Golovina IS. Electromagnetic characterization of rectangular ferroelectric resonators. Journal of Magnetic Resonance. 2005;**174**:292

[82] Geifman IN, Golovina IS. Optimization of ferroelectric resonators for enhanced EPR sensitivity. Concepts in Magenetic Resonance. 2005;**26B**:46

[83] Golovina I, Geifman I, Belous A. New ceramic EPR resonators with high dielectric permittivity. Journal of Magnetic Resonance. 2008;**195**:52

[84] Torrezan AC, Mayer Alegre TP, Medeiros-Ribeiro G. Microstrip resonators for electron paramagnetic resonance experiments. Review of Scientific Instruments. 2009;**80**:044702

[85] Golovina IS, Kolesnik SP, Geifman IN, Belous AG. Novel multisample dielectric resonators for electron paramagnetic resonance spectroscopy. Review of Scientific Instruments. 2010;**81**:044702